Oliver Wendell Holmes in Paris

Becoming Modern: New Nineteenth-Century Studies

SERIES EDITORS

Sarah Way Sherman
Department of English
University of New Hampshire

Janet Aikins
Department of English
University of New Hampshire

Rohan McWilliam
Anglia Ruskin University
Cambridge, England

Janet Polasky
Department of History
University of New Hampshire

This book series maps the complexity of historical change and assesses the forma-tion of ideas, movements, and institutions crucial to our own time by publishing books that examine the emergence of modernity in North America and Europe. Set primarily but not exclusively in the nineteenth century, the series shifts atten-tion from modernity's twentieth-century forms to its earlier moments of uncer-tain and often disputed construction. Seeking books of interest to scholars on both sides of the Atlantic, it thereby encourages the expansion of nineteenth-century studies and the exploration of more global patterns of development.

For a complete list of books in this series, see www.upne.com

Oliver Wendell Holmes in Paris

Medicine, Theology, and
The Autocrat of the Breakfast Table

William C. Dowling

University of New Hampshire
Durham, New Hampshire

PUBLISHED BY

UNIVERSITY PRESS OF NEW ENGLAND

HANOVER AND LONDON

University of New Hampshire Press

Published by University Press of New England,

One Court Street, Lebanon, NH 03766

www.upne.com

© 2006 by University of New Hampshire Press

Printed in the United States of America

5 4 3 2 1

LIBRARY OF CONGRESS CATALOGING-IN-PUBLICATION DATA

Dowling, William C.

Oliver Wendell Holmes in Paris : medicine, theology, and the
Autocrat of the breakfast table / William C. Dowling.

p. ;   cm. — (Becoming modern)

Includes bibliographical references and index.

ISBN-13: 978–1–58465–579–4 (cloth : alk. paper)

ISBN-10: 1–58465–579–8 (cloth : alk. paper)

ISBN-13: 978–1–58465–580–0 (pbk. : alk. paper)

ISBN-10: 1–58465–580–1 (pbk. : alk. paper)

1. Holmes, Oliver Wendell, 1809–1894. 2. Physicians—United States—Biography.
[DNLM: 1. Holmes, Oliver Wendell, 1809–1894. 2. Holmes, Oliver Wendell, 1809–1894.
Autocrat of the breakfast table. 3. Physicians—Biography. 4. Health Knowledge,
Attitudes, Practice. 5. History, 19th Century. 6. Medicine in Literature. 7. Physicians—
history. 8. Religion and Medicine. WZ 100 H752D 2006] I. Title. II. Series.

R154.H636D69   2006

610'.92—dc22   2006001968

For

Loring Conant, M.D.

medicus, amicus, vir iustus

Contents

Preface

The first number of *The Atlantic Monthly* appeared in Boston in November, 1857. The new magazine was the voice of a New England literary culture previously heard only faintly and sporadically in such periodicals as *The Monthly Anthology* and *The North American Review*. Now it was as though, some magic spell having suddenly been broken, it was being permitted to speak in its full strength. By common consent, the single most engaging voice in its pages was that of Oliver Wendell Holmes, a contributor in whom could already be recognized "one of the most brilliant and versatile conversationalists of modern time—the Autocrat of the Breakfast-Table, one who 'invented a new kind in literature,'— a combination of poetry, psychical introspection, and practical philosophy, irradiated by delicate wit, gay humor, and irresistible drollery."[1] "The reader of the *Atlantic*," said Francis H. Underwood, "always turned to the 'Autocrat' first."[2] Throughout the early years of *The Atlantic*, and then after the Civil War in its resumption in *The Poet at the Breakfast Table*, Holmes's breakfast table series would remain the monthly favorite of *Atlantic* readers.

Nor was this true only of American readers. From London, Holmes's close friend John Lothrop Motley delightedly reported on a dinner party at which he had been seated near William Makepeace Thackeray, the celebrated *Punch* satirist and author of *Vanity Fair*. "'Have you read the Autocrat of the Breakfast-Table by Holmes in the new *Atlantic* magazine?'," Thackeray had asked the dining companion across from him. Motley continues: "He then went on to observe that *no man in England* could now write with that charming mixture of wit, pathos and imagination—that your papers were better by far than anything in their magazines."[3] This was not simply the Thackeray of *The Yellowplush Papers* and *Vanity Fair*, but the lecturer and literary critic whose *English Humourists* had made him an acknowledged expert on the tradition of English wit and humor. In Thackeray's dinner-table remarks *The Autocrat of the Breakfast Table* was being judged and found worthy according to a standard set by such English writers as Addison, Fielding, Sterne, and Goldsmith.

Yet it was not only their witty exuberance that won the Breakfast Table books a loyal readership. Throughout his literary career Holmes would get letters—"I have thanked . . . thousands," he says in a late preface, "and many thousands of these kind correspondents."[4]— expressing deep gratitude for the spiritual comfort they had given readers. So, for instance, from Birmingham, England, one Ernest T. Phipson, who had come across the trilogy when "in a state of great depression": "your books were . . . the source of incalculable enjoyment and delight." It must be pleasing to an author, remarked Phipson, to know that "thousands of men and women in all parts of the world . . . are lastingly the better and the happier for what he has written."[5] From Eastbourne, England, Winifred Parnell: "There are not many great modern authors whose works are calculated to make young people feel happy and hopeful."[6] From Edinburgh, Patrick J. Stirling Boyd, thanking Holmes for his "healthy and invigorating thoughts": "as I approached the end, I carefully portioned out the pages, as one would deal out the last handful of bread in a famished city."[7] Or, from America, Laura Brownell Collier, sending to Supreme Court Justice Oliver Wendell Holmes, Jr., a copy of a letter written to her by his father when she was a student at Vassar: "The 'Autocrat,' 'Professor' and 'Poet' were my joy. It seemed as if their author could understand and answer my troubled questionings." [8]

In such letters we glimpse the uneasy stirrings of what we have learned to recognize as Victorian religious anxiety, a deep misery of mind or spirit less psychological—what we should today call clinical depression—than existential: a lived experience of the bleak sense of meaninglessness that sets in when one has awakened to find oneself living in a blind physical universe utterly oblivious to mind or spirit or imagination. The story of its origins in the nineteenth-century triumph of the physical sciences— Lyell's *Elements of Geology* or Darwin's *Origin of Species*, along with such manifestos as Comte's *Cours de philosophie positive*—is a twice told tale. It has seldom been more memorably expressed than by Sainte-Beuve in a passage Holmes copied into one of his notebooks: "Groan over it or not, as we may, Faith has disappeared. Science, let people say what they will, has destroyed it. It is absolutely impossible for vigorous, sensible minds, conversant with history, armed with criticism, studious of the natural sciences, any longer to believe in old stories and old Bibles. So let us men and women cease to be children as soon as possible; this will be a hard task to a great many women—and to a great many men too."[9]

The source of Sainte-Beuve's anguish is less science as such than the doctrines of scientific materialism that had been proclaimed in the later eighteenth century in works like Holbach's *Système de la nature*. These same materialist doctrines are what the philosopher Henry Sidgwick would have in mind in speaking, in Sainte-Beuve's own time, of "atheis-

tic science," meaning something purely neutral and descriptive, a simple recognition that the universe brought into view in Newton's *Principia* in the seventeenth century seemed every day more obviously to be nothing more than a blind whirl of matter governed by purely physical laws. Yet the consequences for religious believers were devastating. Victorian "atheistic science" seemed to leave as the only rational alternative to religious belief an uncompromising materialism that explained away human consciousness and its customary preoccupations—art, religion, morality, logic, mathematics, philosophy, even scientific theories themselves—as mere epiphenomena of matter in its endless combinations. It was this materialism that weighed like a nightmare, as Thomas Henry Huxley sombrely remarked, on many of the best minds of the nineteenth century: "The advancing tide of matter threatens to drown their souls; the tightening grasp of law impedes their freedom; they are alarmed lest man's moral nature be debased by the increase of his wisdom."[10]

This is the background against which Oliver Wendell Holmes's Paris medical studies in the early 1830s assume so crucial an importance, not simply for an understanding of the Breakfast Table series but of Victorian intellectual culture as a whole. For the clinical studies into which Holmes entered at the École de Médecine had their origin in precisely the sort of scientific materialism associated with eighteenth-century philosophes like Helvetius and Holbach, and, perhaps most significantly, with La Mettrie's *L'homme machine*—'man as a machine'—written by a physician who had studied at Leyden with the famous Boerhaave. By the time Holmes arrived in Paris, the notion of medicine as a pursuit solidly grounded in the achievements of modern physics and chemistry was well established. Medicine, the Paris clinical researcher J.B. Bouillaud could declare in 1836, has now "definitively constituted itself on the same bases as the other physical sciences, and . . . will have the right from now on to figure among the exact sciences."[11] In such pronouncements we hear insistent echoes of La Mettrie's conception of the human body as a physical system answering to the same laws as the rest of the physical universe.

The problem posed by Holmes's studies at the École de Médecine turns on an apparent paradox. Holmes departed for Paris at a moment when Lyell's *Elements of Geology* had only recently appeared, counterposing to the Biblical account of Creation a compelling and disturbing argument in favor of millions of years of evolutionary time. Having absorbed the lessons of his Paris teachers, as well as those suggested by the zoological exhibits at the Jardin des Plantes—human and primate skeletons ranged side by side in museum cabinets, silently pointing to what already seemed to many thoughtful observers an obvious conclusion—Holmes would return from Paris with a lifelong allegiance to the views later to be associated in the popular mind with works like Chambers's *Vestiges of Creation* and Darwin's *Origin of Species*. As an author, Holmes would declare that "Parisian" allegiance in such works as *Mechanism in Thought and Morals*. As a teacher, he would do so by constantly reminding his Harvard medical students that the doctor who comes to the bedside, no matter how religious he may personally be, is solely concerned with the anatomico-pathological basis of disease, that "no doctrine of prayer or special providence is to be his excuse for not looking straight at secondary causes."[12] Yet for all his unwavering allegiance to "atheistic science"—this is the apparent paradox—Holmes would never forsake an essentially theological perspective on the problem of human existence.

The solution to the paradox is that Holmes's own studies at the École de Médecine would suggest to him that atheism was only one possible conclusion among others that could be just as legitimately drawn from the new scientific materialism. The alternative view to which he would then commit himself as a writer—based on the *vis medicatrix naturae* and what I shall be calling Holmes's metaphysics of consciousness—began in the new conception of diagnosis and disease that originated in Xavier Bichat's brilliant researches in tissue pathology at the Hôtel Dieu in Paris, which rendered instantly obsolete the older humoral conception of disease that had dominated medicine from the time of Hippocrates and Galen to the end of the eighteenth century. Bichat's *Anatomie générale* (1801) had brought into view an interior world of the body demanding an entirely new conception of disease as an autonomous entity, a break with Galenic or traditional medicine so profound as to be termed by historians of Paris medicine an epistemological rupture (*coupure*).[13] Bichat's approach to pathology was based on what was then termed *solidism* and *localism*, solidism being the doctrine that diseases originated in solid organs like the kidneys or heart, as opposed to the humoral fluids, localism the doctrine that disease was due not to some general derangement of humoral balance but to local alterations in a tissue or organ.

The immense achievement represented by Bichat's *Anatomie générale* rested upon thousands of post mortem dissections. As Bichat famously said, a physician could spend twenty years taking bedside notes on the obscure outward symptoms of diseases of the heart, lungs, and stomach, but "open a few corpses, and immediately this obscurity, which observation alone would never have removed, will disappear."[14] Paris alone of European cities in the earlier nineteenth century offered medical students unlimited opportunities to dissect. As John Harley Warner's magisterial *Against the Spirit of System* has shown, it was overwhelmingly the opportunity to pursue unlimited anatomico-pathological studies at the École Pratique d'Anatomie and the famous dissecting amphitheater at Clamart that drew American students like Holmes to Paris. Four thousand corpses annually, one American medical student would delightedly report, were collected from the hospitals and delivered to the École Pratique and the Clamart:

> Every day, at twelve o'clock, there is a distribution of them among all the classes of students. Every instructor has a small building for his own use, in which are ten or fifteen tables of cast iron. The human body may thus be viewed in every stage of dissection, and, I may add, decomposition. By perambulating the several buildings, the various parts of the human organism, the nerves, muscles and blood-vessels may be easily examined, and studied. Here, the assiduous student may be seen, with his soiled blouse, and his head bedecked with a fantastic cap. In one hand he holds a scalpel, in the other a treatise on anatomy.[15]

The epistemological break separating Paris clinical teaching from the older humoral medicine occurred largely with the walls of a single Paris institution, the Hospital of La Charité.[16] In its wards, a group of researchers so distinct as to become spoken of as the School of La Charité would arrive at a new notion of disease as an autonomous entity. The work of three men in particular would influence Holmes. The first was Jean Nicholas Corvisart, who in rediscovering the technique of percussion—tapping or thumping the chest to determine the state of the organs within—found an external means of exploring the interior world of the body brought into view by Bichat's anatomico-pathological discoveries. The second was René Théophile Hyacinthe Laennec, inventor of the stethoscope. Laennec's invention permitted the trained diagnostician to identify the distinct pathological states associated with specific stages of a particular disease, a famous example being the cavities in the tissue of the lung—"tubercular excavations"—that were the sign of advanced tuberculosis. It was specifically Laennec's method of stethoscopic diagnosis that Holmes was recalling, for instance, when he spoke in a Boylston Prize essay written immediately after his return from Paris of "that wonderful art of discovering disease, which, as it were, puts a window in the breast, through which the vital organs can be seen."[17]

Laennec's invention of the stethoscope is a vivid example of what historians of Paris medicine mean by the epistemological rupture associated with *l'école de La Charité*. The new methods of diagnosis did not simply mark a new way of correlating external symptoms with internal pathological states. They represented as well a sharp break with fifteen centuries of what Jacalyn Duffin has called subjective symptomology: the idea that to be sick, and especially sick enough to call a doctor, one had to *feel* sick.[18] Today, when CAT scans and MRIs routinely reveal the presence of deadly disease in patients who feel themselves to be in robust good health, it is hard to imagine a time when this could count as a revolutionary idea. In the Paris in which Holmes arrived in 1833, its revolutionary implications were at once obvious and unsettling. For the first time in history, diagnosis was putting physicians in possession of knowledge—in many cases, of life-or-death knowledge—unknown to their patients. Holmes's later battle against such forms of medical quackery as homeopathy began in his conviction, brought home from his Paris studies, that such knowledge was the only valid basis of medical practice, and would inevitably be increased by systematic scientific investigation.

The third great medical researcher at La Charité to influence Holmes would do so in personal as well as scientific terms. This was Pierre Charles Alexandre Louis, a modest and retiring clinical investigator whose influence on Holmes's group of Boston medical students was so enormous as to make him in effect the tutelary spirit of New England medicine for the next half-century. By the time Holmes arrived in Paris, Louis had already earned an international reputation for his studies of tuberculosis (then called *phthisis*, from a Greek term describing a slow wasting away) and typhoid fever. Louis's reputation rested on his "numerical method." In an age so far largely innocent of what we should now call clinical statistics, Louis was the first serious medical researcher to compile painstaking and systematic numerical tables relating the incidence of disease to such variables as age, sex, occupation, and family medical history, to record the ordinary duration of common illnesses, the percentages of favorable versus unfavorable outcomes, and, in cases permitting autopsy, to track the relation of external symptoms to internal pathological alterations over the entire course of a disease.

For the young American physicians of Holmes's generation, the great importance of Louis's numerical method lay in its challenge to long-established therapeutic doctrines. They had come to Paris from an America in which bloodletting, normally by venesection, was the normal procedure in scores of diseases and conditions, and in which massive bloodletting had been authorized by such celebrated teachers as Benjamin Rush. (Up to four-fifths of the blood could be removed from the body without danger, we will hear Rush rashly and erroneously telling his students, adding reassuringly that " 'Tis a very hard matter to bleed a patient to death.") In his *Recherches sur les effets de la saignée*—translated into English as *Researches on the Effects of Bloodletting in Some Inflammatory Diseases*—Louis conclusively demonstrated that bloodletting either had no effect on diseases or, in a number of cases, made them worse. In the eyes of the Boston students who had studied with him in Paris, Louis's monumental achievement had been to show by rigorous statistical analysis that bleeding did not shorten the course of acute diseases like pneumonia, for which venesection had long been a standard remedy.

"This was not a reform," Holmes would tell his class of Harvard medical students, "—it was a revolution."[19]

The medical perspective for which Holmes is speaking was called "therapeutic skepticism," or, by its most vociferous opponents, therapeutic nihilism. In its name, Holmes and other New England physicians would challenge the bleeding, purging, drugging practice that had been carried on for centuries as the main legacy of Galenic medicine. As promulgated by physicians like Benjamin Rush, this was called "heroic" practice, implying that in cases when a patient had become seriously ill, the doctor must take audacious measures to save the patient from his mortal enemy. In illness, Rush would solemnly tell his class of American medical students, that enemy was Nature itself. By contrast, the Parisian school centered in Boston and led by students of Louis—the school for which Holmes became a major spokesman—was known for its uncompromising opposition to heroic practice. "The disgrace of medicine," Holmes would say in one of his Harvard lectures, "has been that colossal system of self-deception, in obedience to which mines have been emptied of their cankering minerals, the vegetable kingdom robbed of all its noxious growths, the entrails of animals taxed for their impurities, the poison-bags of reptiles drained of their venom, and all the inconceivable abominations thus obtained thrust down the throats of human beings."[20]

The alternative to heroic practice was the Parisian *méthode expectante* or "expectant method": palliative care meant to aid nature in her spontaneous attempts to bring about recovery. In Paris, the *méthode expectante* was taken to be a therapeutic doctrine only. In Boston, Oliver Wendell Holmes, having recognized that there lay at the core of the *méthode expectante* an essentially metaphysical conception of the impulse toward regeneration in the living body, would come to see in the *vis medicatrix naturae*—the healing power of nature, with "power" still carrying archaic or classical associations with a higher agency—intimations of a divine principle at work in the universe of living beings. As a Harvard professor of anatomy and physiology, Holmes was an omnivorous reader of the newest medical literature arriving from France and, later, Germany. In the years after Virchow's groundbreaking researches in cell biology, especially, he would come to regard modern scientific medicine more and more as a detailed revelation of the *vis medicatrix*. Yet he would also find himself moving inexorably toward a vision of science itself as the modern form of revelation, as we hear in his description of the new compound microscope that had made Virchow's discoveries possible:

These wonderful discoveries which we owe to that mighty little instrument, the telescope of the inner firmament with all its included worlds;

those simple formulae by which we condense the observations of a generation in a single axiom . . . all lead us up to the inspiration of the Almighty,
which gives understanding to the world's great teachers. To fear science
or knowledge, lest it disturb our old beliefs, is to fear the influx of the
Divine wisdom into the souls of our fellow-men; for what is science but the
piecemeal *revelation*,—uncovering,—of the plan of creation, by the agency
of those chosen prophets of nature whom God has illuminated from the
central light of truth for that single purpose?[21]

As the revelation of a benign or benevolent purpose at work in the
universe, the *vis medicatrix* would become for Holmes the very antidote
to the Calvinist doctrines—the angry God of Jonathan Edwards, Innate
Depravity, the predestination of human souls to eternal torment—that lay
at the heart of New England theology. For in light of his medical studies,
the vengeful God of Calvinism had come to seem to Holmes not a real
deity but a gigantic and monstrous projection of the darkest impulses in
human moral nature. The Calvinist doctrine of predestination, in particular, seemed to him to posit a God who derived enjoyment "from the
infliction of misery on sensitive beings, who, by the fact of coming into
existence under conditions provided or permitted by their Creator, have
incurred his wrath and received his curse as their patrimony."[22] Hatred
of Calvinism—it is not too strong a word—was still largely a repressed
or unexpressed sentiment in the young Holmes who departed for Paris
only a few years after his graduation from Harvard. For the Holmes who
returned from his decisive years in Paris to embark upon his career as a
physician, professor of medicine, and medical writer, by contrast, Calvinism had become a derangement of the moral imagination amounting to
a spiritual disease.

When Holmes speaks of scientists like Virchow as prophets of nature,
on the other hand, or of medical discoveries as illuminations of a divinely-
revealed truth, we glimpse the underlying metaphysics of consciousness
that gave his Breakfast Table trilogy so great a power of spiritual reassur-
ance for nineteenth-century readers. In the trilogy as a whole, this power
emerges only gradually. When James Russell Lowell recruited Holmes as
a contributor to the newly-founded *Atlantic Monthly*, the man he hoped
to enlist was the Holmes of the Saturday Club, the famously witty conver-
sationalist and clever versifier ready for any occasion. "Lowell was never
tired of saying," William Dean Howells would recall, that "the magazine
could never have gone at all without the Autocrat papers."[23] Long before
the *Autocrat* had arrived at its last installment, however, a markedly different Holmesian persona would have emerged at the boarding-house
breakfast table: a deeper, more serious speaker whose brilliant wit had
become a weapon turned at once against the grim universe of Calvin-

ist theology and the bleak materialism of the French Enlightenment. A contemporary biographer, W. S. Kennedy, was among to the first to note this deeper, less familiar Holmes, glimpsing beyond the "humorous poet and satirico-humorous essayist" of the Breakfast Table trilogy "a lay-preacher, an earnest thinker, a cultured and accurate teacher, and an original scientific investigator."[24]

This is Holmes as physician of the spirit in an age of deep religious anxiety. In *The Professor at the Breakfast Table*, the Professor is a member of the faculty at a famous medical school, a physician whose simultaneous interest in science and theology channels the flow of conversation throughout. In the third volume of the trilogy, *The Poet at the Breakfast Table*, the spokesman for scientific truth as inspired wisdom will be "the Master," a learned polymath whose fascinated interest in Darwin and evolution, Pasteur and germ theory, and the ongoing revelations of geology and paleontology—"Those new tables of the law, placed in the hands of the geologist by the same living God who spoke from Sinai to the Israelites of old," as Holmes calls them[25]—will lead him to proclaim the *vis medicatrix* and the metaphysics of rational consciousness as a new gospel of hope and reconciliation. Yet as Holmes makes clear at the end of the trilogy, the Autocrat, the Professor, and the Poet have been a single voice throughout, belonging to a man who has looked into himself only to discover a microcosm of humanity as a whole.[26] "He sought the universal through himself in others," W.D Howells would say.[27] In doing so, as we shall see, Holmes would emerge as the spiritual physician of his own time, offering to readers throughout the English-speaking world a *religio medici* meant for the modern age.

A number of people provided invaluable aid during the research and writing of *Oliver Wendell Holmes in Paris*. In particular, I'd like to thank the staff of Houghton Library for their patience over the long series of summers that it took to learn my way around the Holmes repository. In Paris, the staff of the Bibliothèque of the École de Médecine was similarly patient with an American visitor given only a single semester's research leave to master the nineteenth-century French medical writings essential to reconstructing the context of Holmes's studies. At the Countway Medical Library, Thomas Horrocks was especially resourceful in helping me track down materials relating to the impact of Paris medicine on Boston physicians. I'm grateful to them all.

To a number of particular individuals, I owe a debt beyond gratitude. Tom and Vera Kreilkamp provided me with a home away from home during the summers I was working at Houghton and the Countway Library. Without that timely support, the book couldn't have been written. Sherwin B. Nuland and Jacalyn Duffin, both physicians and distinguished historians of medicine, took time out from crowded schedules to answer technical questions about nineteenth-century anatomy, physiology, and pathology. My friend and neighbor Michael Ruddy, also a physician and professor of medicine, allowed himself to be badgered with detailed questions about cell biology, neurotransmitters, and the semantics of modern disease classification. Mark Schaeffer, my personal physician, was especially helpful in the early period when I was doing my best to grasp the content of Holmes's anatomy lectures at Harvard Medical School.

As for the actual writing, two people are responsible for the present version of *Oliver Wendell Holmes in Paris*: Linda Dowling, whose concentrated work on the medical chapters permitted them to emerge as something like a coherent narrative, and Phyllis Deutsch, senior editor at the University Press of New England, who began by insisting that the two final chapters situate Holmes more intelligibly in Victorian intellectual culture, and who then walked me through the series of revisions from which—as I may perhaps be permitted to hope—a final illumination was to dawn. A book some years ago about the great Max Perkins at Scribners bore the title *Editor of Genius*. I had two of them. Every scholar should be so lucky.

Oliver Wendell Holmes in Paris

CHAPTER ONE

The Discovery of Disease

On November 28, 1882, Dr. Oliver Wendell Holmes made a final appearance before his class at Harvard Medical school, the course in anatomy he had been teaching since becoming Parkman Professor of Anatomy and Physiology in 1847. He had intended to give his usual lecture and then say an informal word of farewell to his students, but finding that something more was expected from the author of *The Autocrat of the Breakfast Table* and other well-known works, and that numerous visitors would be attending this last class, he spent the previous evening putting together notes for a final address. It was a reminiscence, full of the acerbic wit and genial wisdom for which Holmes was so well known as an author, of his own days as a medical student nearly fifty years earlier. It was later published in his *Medical Essays* under the title "Some of My Early Teachers."

For the most part, Holmes's reminiscence concerns his study in Paris, during a revolution in medical theory and clinical teaching that had already passed into legend by the time he was addressing this final class. When thinking about possible topics for these last remarks, Holmes tells them, it occurred to him that they "may like to hear something of the famous Professors of Paris in the days when I was a student in the École de Médecine, and following the great hospital teachers."[1] His talk is a vivid recollection of days spent in the hospitals and clinics and lecture rooms to which Erwin Ackerknecht, its first great historian, referred as "the Paris hospital," meaning the entire system of research and teaching institutions within which the conceptual foundations of modern scientific medicine were laid down.

In Holmes's last lecture, the great teachers of his Paris days come alive as the vivid personalities they were, holding forth not only before French students, but multitudes drawn from every corner of Europe, as well as from America and Russia and Africa, to follow the great hospital teachers on their rounds. There is Broussais, spluttering like an ancient volcano now that his famous theory of enteric inflammation is widely regarded as having been disproved, and Velpeau, the peasant boy from the provinces who has risen to the top of Parisian surgery by talent and unremitting industry, and Pierre Charles Alexandre Louis, whose invention of the "numerical system" of correlating external symptoms with internal lesions would not only revolutionize medical theory but provide a new basis of medical practice for the singularly brilliant group of American students—James Jackson, Jr., Jonathan Mason Warren, Henry I. Bowditch, Holmes himself—who lived and studied together in Paris during this period.

At the end of his remarks, Holmes runs off a list of figures who even by the time he is speaking have become mere footnotes in the history of medicine: "where is Civiale," he asks rhetorically, "—where are Orfila, Genrin, Rostan, Biett, Alibert?"[2] In the days when Holmes was actually studying in Paris, these names would have been instantly recognizable to anyone current with modern medical teaching. Civiale, for instance, was especially prominent because he had invented a procedure that solved the problem of removing bladder stones without invasive surgery, thus sparing numberless patients, in the days before anesthesia, an agonizing operation and the strong likelihood of death from postoperative infection. A modest and amiable man, he grew wealthy on the fees he earned from performing his operation, as patients ranging from ordinary burghers to princes traveled from the most distant parts of Europe to avoid the danger of subjecting themselves to a local surgeon.

As it happens, some of the most detailed accounts of Civiale's operation available to us occur in letters written home by one of Holmes's Boston friends, a medical student who was already completing his own first year in Paris when Holmes arrived in early May, 1833. This was Jonathan Mason Warren—called "Mason" by his family and friends—the scion of a famous Massachusetts medical family. He was the son of John Collins Warren, a leading surgeon and professor of medicine who had been Holmes's own teacher of anatomy and physiology at Harvard. Mason Warren's letters to his physician father are among the most vivid and exact records we have of Paris medicine during the period Holmes studied there. Mason's description of Civiale's procedure is representative:

Civiale commenced the operation by introducing a small catheter and injected about a pint of warm water into the bladder. The catheter was then withdrawn and the *brise-pierre* well-oiled was introduced slowly and slipped into the bladder with the greatest ease. The jaws of the instrument were now opened and the stone sought for. This being found the jaws were closed and the drill forced tight down upon it. A handle was

Oliver Wendell Holmes in Paris

now added to the instrument, it being steadied by an assistant. The drill was turned rapidly with the bow and the stone broken. . . . The operation lasted about ten minutes and was all done with no pain except from the retention of the water.[3]

The crucial elements of Civiale's procedure can be gotten from Mason's description. It was called *lithotrity*, to distinguish it from the standard operation of *lithotomy*, or, as it was popularly called by physicians and patients alike, "cutting for the stone." Its genius lay in the instrument Civiale had invented, what medical historians call a "trilabe" and Mason calls the *brise-pierre*, or "stone crusher." This was a metal cylinder that could be inserted through the urethra, the membranous channel that runs through the penis to the bladder. Within it was concealed a three-jawed instrument that could, by partially withdrawing the outer cylinder, be opened inside the bladder. The three jaws were then clamped down on the stone, a drill inserted through the center of the inner cylinder, and the stone broken into fragments. In the ideal case, these fragments would be small enough to be passed in the urine. In the more normal case, repeated operations could be undertaken on the larger fragments, until all were passed.

In our own age of anesthesia and antibiotics, it is virtually impossible to imagine the relief from fear and anxiety that Civiale's operation brought to thousands of sufferers from the stone. Some sense of how revolutionary it was can be gotten from the remarks of Valentine Mott, himself a famous American surgeon and professor at Rutgers Medical School, after a visit made to Paris in 1835. At the Hospital of Necker, reports Mott, "resides the ever-illustrious and unrivaled Civiale, the projector and the author of that greatest of all triumphs for science and humanity, . . . the operation of *lithotrity*. How much pain, how much agony, has not this great and good man saved to his fellow-creatures!" Civiale's victory has been, as Mott properly says, "over one of the most afflicting and excruciating torments which it is the lot of mortals to endure." His wondering remarks at Civiale's operative technique are high praise from one accomplished surgeon to another: "in his speciality, of all the men I have ever seen, for delicacy of tact and adroitness of execution he surpasses. It is utterly impossible for any one to imagine the highly finished style of his manipulations."[4]

The setting in which Mason Warren was watching Civiale perform his operation was the scene of a revolution against the Galenic medicine that had dominated western theory and practice for centuries. This was, famously, a medicine based on the theory of the four humors, bodily fluids corresponding to the four elements (earth, air, fire, water) that in the ancient world had been considered the ultimate constituents of all material bodies. In the later middle ages, when Paris first emerged as a world center of medical teaching, Galenic medicine had already dominated clinical theory for nearly a thousand years: "The humors—phlegm, blood, bile, and black bile—were cold and moist, hot and moist, hot and dry, and cold and dry, respectively," writes one medieval historian, describing Paris medicine in the twelfth century. "These qualities were the complexions of the humors. All drugs of the pharmacopoeia were classified according to their degrees of moisture, dryness, heat, and cold, and they were prescribed so as to maintain the proper balance of the humors within the body. The physician 'discovered' how these were out of balance by examining visually the urine, sometimes the stool, and by feeling the pulse of the right wrist."[5]

In his own medical writings, Holmes would very often stress the sense in which Galenic theory imagined the human body as a microcosm of the physical universe, the balance of humors that constituted health corresponding to the proportion of elements in the external world. "Its theory," wrote Holmes in one of his numerous accomplished essays in the history of medicine, "was that the body, the microcosm, like the macrocosm, was made up of the four elements—fire, air, water, earth, having respectively the qualities hot, dry, moist, cold. The body was to be preserved in health by keeping each of these qualities in its natural proportion; heat, by the proper temperature; moisture, by the due amount of fluid; and so as to the rest. Diseases which arose from excess of heat were to be attacked by cooling remedies; those from excess of cold, by heating ones, and so of the other derangements of balance." The Galenic physician, Holmes adds, "attributed the four fundamental qualities to different vegetables, in four different degrees; thus chicory was cold in the fourth degree, pepper was hot in the fourth. . . .When we say 'Cool as a cucumber,' we are talking Galenism."[6]

In the immediate background of Holmes's remarks to his final Harvard class lay, as well, another survival of older medical theory that would come to be exploded during his own time in Paris. This was *nosology*, or the systematic classification of symptoms by type and degree. In general terms, nosology was an expression of the same impulse of Enlightenment rationalism by which Linnaeus revolutionized the study of animal and plant life through a taxonomy of genus and species. The problem was that eighteenth-century nosology then tended to identify "disease" with an appropriately classified constellation of symptoms. The most famous example is Philippe Pinel, whose *Nosographie philosophique* (1798) provided an elaborate system of classification the major weakness of which was, as Erwin Ackerknecht says, that symptoms were again and again "elevated to the rank of disease units": "Worst in this respect was . . . his first class, 'essential fevers' . . . It is legitimate that it has been criticized most severely. Many of our present units, such as typhoid fever, malaria, or diphtheria, occur in several of his subdivisions and cannot be identified with any one of them."[7]

In general terms, Pinel's *Nosographie* may be regarded as just another of the systems that would be exploded by Pasteur and germ theory at the end of the nineteenth century. For students of the Paris medical revolution, however, its value lies in the final illumination it casts on a concept of disease that, at a deeper level, had underwritten medical theory for centuries. For the phenomenon of what Jacalyn Duffin has called "subjective symptomology" had been the underlying basis of medical theory since the days of Hippocrates and Galen: "When confronted with a patient having a certain combination of symptoms evolving in a certain sequence, astute observers would be able to apply a name to the patient's condition. . . . To make a diagnosis, the patient's history—the subjective account of the illness—was of paramount importance. Physical signs—derived from the pulse, touching, and observation of skin and excreta—were of lesser importance. In the eighteenth century, a physical disease was not an anatomical object, it was a physiological event; for its recognition, the patient was the final arbiter."[8]

Up to the very end of the eighteenth century, in short, "disease" was conceivable only as a sensation of illness immediately perceived by the patient, and only secondarily or inferentially diagnosable by the physician. " A person could not be sick," as Duffin puts it, "without feeling sick."[9] By the middle of the nineteenth century, on the other hand, disease could be conceptualized as a separate entity that might well have taken up residence in the body without the patient's being aware of it. Today, when people routinely take medication for deadly but symptomless conditions like high blood pressure, and when all are tremulously aware that cancer might be silently developing anywhere in the body, this conception scarcely seems revolutionary. Yet this new and alternative conception of disease was the basis of the revolution in medical theory that drew students like Warren and Holmes to Paris. No one has written about it better than Duffin, whose superb study of René Théophile Hyacinthe Laennec, the inventor of the stethoscope, isolates the very moment of reversal. With Laennec's invention, writes Duffin, it was finally possible "for physicians to prove that a person was physically sick without feeling sick. With the stethoscope, the doctor could detect a lesion before the patient had suffered any symptoms. Even people who felt completely well could no longer be certain that they were. Reiser compared Laennec's invention to Gutenberg's, as the instrument that turned the focus of medicine from sick people to disease. Physicians became the custodians of knowledge that had previously belonged only to their patients."[10]

The Paris medical revolution, however, though it would ultimately produce a wholly new concept of disease, originated primarily as an attack on a mode of training associated in France with the *ancien régime*, one that had remained essentially unchanged for centuries. Though there were variations among the European countries—Leyden, Bologna, and Padua were known as centers of "progressive" theory—the basic principle of traditional training had since medieval times been a ritualistic exposition of Galenic theory, which by necessity placed a high value on knowledge of Greek and Latin. A representative version of the traditional regimen was that obtaining in eighteenth-century Oxford: "To receive the degree of doctor of medicine at Oxford originally required fourteen years attendance at the university: four years for the bachelor of arts, three more for the master of arts, three more for the bachelor of medicine, and four more for the doctor of medicine. . . . The medical education was largely a study of the ancient authors; the examinations for the doctor's degree required an explanation of a whole book of Galen in six extemporaneous lectures or three written lectures. To such an extent had this gone that Sydenham is said to have declared that medicine was not to be learned by going to universities."[11]

The Parisian reaction against this mode of medical training was part of the wave of radical ideas that swept through France after the storming of the Bastille in 1789: not simply new doctrines of liberty and equality but a surfacing of the philosophical materialism that remained an unacknowledged or underground discourse during the years of the *ancien régime*. As Ackerknecht's *Medicine in the Paris Hospital* shows, the universe out of which the new Paris medicine would emerge was not least the universe of La Mettrie's *L'homme machine*, written by a Boerhaave-trained physician who dared to argue that a human being was just another physical system in the physical universe, or Holbach's *Système de la nature*, with its unflinching picture of the universe as, in the words of James Boswell, the biographer of Samuel Johnson, "an eternal necessity without design." This was the unrepentant atheism and materialism of the French Enlightenment at its most radical, a strain of thought that would exert a profound influence on Parisian thinking at least until the fall of Robespierre in 1794.

The radical critique of traditional medical training that emerged from the French Revolution would concentrate on two perceived weaknesses of the older system: it existed in isolation from the physical sciences that were taken by the philosophes of the prerevolutionary period to be the glory of Enlightenment rationalism, the strongest evidence possible that humankind in the period since Bacon's *Novum Organon* and Copernicus's *De revolutionibus orbis* had been living in an entirely different conceptual universe than ancient medical writers like Hippocrates and Galen, and it ignored actual patients suffering from actual illnesses in favor of empty theorizing about such matters as plethora and humoral balance. Vicq d'Azyr's polemic against the old system, issued in 1790, is typical: "What can be expected of schools where, in the majority of cases, there is no teaching of either human anatomy in its entirety, or the art of dissection, or botany, or medical chemistry in its full scope, or pharmacy, or the art of writing prescriptions, or nosology, or the history of medicine, or pathology; where not one word is said of the public functions of medicine; where no one has taught his art at the bedside of the sick?"[12]

The succession of events that would end in the radical reorganization of the Paris hospital system, putting Paris medical teaching, Holmes would later claim, a half-century ahead of the rest of the world,[13] began with a report submitted to the National Convention by Antoine François Fourcroy in 1794: "It is not sufficient to give lessons and public courses on all branches of science. The old method did not give a complete course and was limited to words. . . . Once the lesson was finished, its contents vanished from the students' memory." In the new École de Santé, wrote Fourcroy—this was temporarily the name of the new Paris medical school—"manipulation will be united with theoretical precepts. The students will do chemical exercises, dissections, operations, and bandaging. *Little reading, much seeing, and much doing will be the foundation of the new teaching which your committee suggests. Practicing the art, observing at the bedside, all that was missing, will now be the principle part of instruction*"[14]

The great advantage given to the reformers was the extensive system of Parisian hospitals that had been founded by various religious orders and private individuals from the Middle Ages onwards, obeying a commandment to charity specifically enjoined by New Testament Christianity and providing care and sustenance for those too poor to be cared for by their own families in times of serious illness. To American students like Holmes and his friends, the medieval setting of their French medical teaching would always be remembered as an important part of their experience, a reminder that Paris had been an international city, and the Latin Quarter, specifically, a magnet for students from other nations, for centuries. To walk the streets of the Latin Quarter was to pass through scenes that had been familiar to international students in the days when Thomas Aquinas and Peter Abelard had drawn crowds to their lectures centuries before.

A setting that would become intimately familiar to both Mason Warren and Holmes, for instance, was the Hôtel Dieu, standing on the Île de la Cité only a few hundred yards from the cathedral of Notre Dame and, in their own time in Paris, joined to a matching wing on the other side of the river. A sense of the timelessness that came over students entering one of the Paris hospitals can be gotten from Augustus Gardner, whose account of his own experience is one of the most valuable sources for those studying American students in Paris during this period: "The oldest hospital in Paris, and, among the first in extent, stands the Hôtel-Dieu. . . . The noble buildings of the Hôtel-Dieu have no claim to architectural elegance, being chiefly remarkable for solidity. The work of several ages, their uncertain origin is attributed to St. Landri, Bishop of Paris in the seventh century. . . . It extends, at present, along both sides of the river Seine, the buildings being united by a tunnel passing under it."[15]

As we shall see, an important element of their Paris experience for Holmes and his friends would be due to a similar sense of having dwelt in a milieu in which the very new—the ethos of Enlightenment rationalism and materialism that had produced the Paris medical revolution—and the very ancient—the Latin Quarter, with its timeless sense of a setting devoted to the pursuit of knowledge for its own sake—imperceptibly blended in their memories of the Paris hospital. For such scenes, as Gardner says elsewhere, are "ever invested with the halo of romance; every object seems enlarged by the mist of ages, with which it is enveloped." Americans, especially, he points out, arriving in Paris from a new civilization only recently won from the wilderness, without ancient traditions and established codes of manners, can hardly help but be struck by the "unequal comparison with the plainness, sometimes even coarseness of their birth-place."[16] For Holmes and his friends, this would be an aspect of their Paris experience that set them apart when they returned to the United States, part of what it means to say that a school of "Parisian" medical thought would develop in America, and particularly in Boston, over the next several decades.

For Parisian medical reformers such as Vicq d'Azyr and Fourcroy, on the other hand, the horror of the hospital system as it had come down from the Middle Ages was that, in an age of population growth and increasing urbanization, it had lost touch with its origins in Christian charity and become little more than a way of warehousing the urban poor, a direct consequence, as Ackerknecht says, "of the tremendous influx of uprooted and penniless boys and girls from the country and of the beginnings of the Industrial Revolution."[17] The result, as well as the proto-Dickensian ferocity it aroused in reformers, survives vividly in the report made by Jacques René Tenon on hospital conditions in 1788, on the very eve of the French Revolution:

The general policy of the Hôtel Dieu—policy caused by the lack of space—is to put as many beds as possible into one room and to put four, five, or six people into one bed. We have seen the dead mixed with the living there. We have seen rooms so narrow that the air stagnates and is not renewed and that light enters only feebly and charged with vapors. We have seen convalescents together with the sick, the dying, and the dead. . . . We have seen a room for convalescents on the third floor, which could be reached only via the small pox ward. . . . Often we saw contagious and noncontagious diseases in the same wards, women with syphilis and some with fever. The operation ward where they trephine, cut the stone, and amputate members contains those who are being operated upon, those who will be operated upon, and those who have already been operated upon.[18]

One paradox of the Paris medical revolution is thus that it began as an anti-hospital movement. In the early days of the Revolution, the conditions described by Tenon led to a general demand for outright abolition of the hospital system. What saved the system was the equal and opposite campaign on the part of men like Fourcroy for medical teaching that would incorporate the advances made during the eighteenth century in sciences like physics and chemistry. They argued forcefully that the existing hospital system, given a radical reorganization, could be remade not only in the interests of humane care but of advances in medical research that would benefit all classes of society. The new medical schools set up by the Convention, urged Fourcroy, must undertake nothing less than a total reconstitution of medical knowledge: "Their function is not to be limited to teaching what is known: they have as their further purpose the most extensive research into all the branches of the art of healing; they have as their aim the advancement of all the sciences which can shed light on the physics of life."[19]

At a practical level, the reorganization of the Paris hospital system would consist of a rededication of specific facilities to specific purposes, as with such specialized hospitals as the Enfants Malades, the first hospital in the world devoted to children's disorders, the Maternité, the lying-in hospital located in the former Port Royal monastery, or the Clamart, the large arena for anatomical dissection in which medical students spent so much of their time. At an administrative level, the reorganization consisted of a new merit-based hierarchy of research and teaching meant to replace the privilege-based order of the *ancien régime*. The dramatic transformation that then occurred was described by Guillaume Dupuytren, the most prominent surgeon in a city of brilliant operators, in a speech given in 1821: "We will remember for a long time the care that was taken in the choice of the masters and students who were supposed to compose these famous schools. From all parts of France they called the most distinguished men and the students who were the most appropriate to benefit from the lessons of such masters."[20]

The heart of the arrangements Dupuytren is talking about, and perhaps their most radical element, was the *concours* system, a public com-
petitive examination through which any candidate might aspire to the
highest position in the hierarchy of hospital teaching. The *concours* was
preeminently, as Ackerknecht says, an expression of the democratic
trends set in motion by the Revolution, a strong reaction against the old
order of privilege and wealth and family connection that had dominated
medical education under the *ancien régime.* In substituting French for
Latin as the language of medical instruction, as Ackerknecht also points
out, it was a direct expression of the nationalistic aspirations that had
been born along with the French Revolution. No longer would a candidate for the medical faculty have to know the languages of Galen and
Celsus to compete for an appointment in anatomy or materia medica. In
purely linguistic terms, the language he shared with his students would
be French. In medical terms, it would be what Russell Maulitz has called
the new "language of the body" developed in the groundbreaking pathological studies of such men as Bichat, Bayle, and Laennec.[21]

Since the *concours* system was developed during the period when the
Napoleonic wars made getting to Paris inordinately difficult for foreign
students, and especially students coming over from an England engaged
in a struggle to the death with Napoleon, very few reports of how the
system worked have come down to us from American medical students
prior to 1815. As it happens, one of these comes from the pen of John
Collins Warren, Mason Warren's father and Holmes's own professor of
anatomy and physiology at Harvard. John Collins Warren had managed
to get to Paris in 1800. His account, written when he was at home in Boston many years later, captures the excitement that surrounded competition for appointments under the *concours*:

> When Dupuytren was first chosen hospital-surgeon, his principal oppo-
> nent was M. Roux, the present distinguished surgeon of the Hôtel Dieu.
> As usual in Paris, a *concours,* or comparative trial of ability, was opened and
> maintained with great skill. I was present at this conflict, which took place
> at the Oratoire, and was astonished at the facility with which the candi-
> dates, on drawing an unknown question from the urn, entered without
> hesitation on a response which extended to a variety of topics branching
> out from the original inquiry. At the end of two days, the balance of opin-
> ion inclined to the side of Roux. Dupuytren had his mind so strongly fixed
> on obtaining the place, that he was almost distracted at the appearance of
> probability in Roux's favor.[22]

When American medical students began to stream into Paris after
Napoleon's defeat at Waterloo, they would almost universally seize upon

the *concours* system as one ideally suited to their own democratic society, in which status in the medical profession was too often anomalously owing, as Augustus Gardner would put it, "to rich relations, or powerful friends." The superiority of the *concours*, he said, was due to the fact that it made "talent, not influence, the necessary requisite for promotion. Every medical office in France, whether military or civil, is thus obtainable by merit. The system extends from the dressers and students in pharmacy up to the professors and highest offices; the qualifications of course increasing with the importance of the place contested." As a shining example of the way the *concours* opened the path to success to even the poorest student, Gardner cites the example of "the celebrated Velpeau, surgeon-in-chief to the hospital *La Charité*."[23]

The personal history of Armand Velpeau, born into a blacksmith's family and at first self-educated, later pursuing his medical education under conditions of barely imaginable penury, would take on an almost allegorical significance for American medical students, including Oliver Wendell Holmes, who as an American author would later, in the age of Jacksonian backwoods democracy, sometimes be accused of an undemocratic or "Federalist" partiality for birth and education. Yet for Holmes, as for Gardner, the *concours* would always remain the symbol of a system that justly rewarded talent and industry over privilege, and Velpeau the emblem of its success. Velpeau's example, Holmes said in the address to students in his last anatomy class, "may be an encouragement to some of my younger hearers who are born, not with the silver spoon in their mouths, but with the two-tined iron fork in their hands. . . . He had not what is called genius, . . . but he had industry, determination, intelligence, character, and he made his way to distinction." "A good sound head over a pair of wooden shoes," concludes Holmes, pointing the moral, "is a great deal better than a wooden head belonging to an owner who cases his feet in calf-skin."[24]

Beyond this reordering of practical arrangements, the conceptual center of the Paris medical revolution lay in that new conception of disease described by Jacalyn Duffin, the epistemological reversal in which illness would go from being something immediately experienced by the patient—the older concept of disease in which, as we have heard Duffin say, "a person could not be sick without feeling sick"—to the notion of disease as an entity harbored within the body and, in many cases, perceptible to the physician even when patients felt perfectly healthy. This was the radically new conception of disease that had originated in Bichat's studies in tissue pathology at the very beginning of Paris medical reorganization, which kept so insistently pointing to internal lesions as the source of the symptoms which might only much later appear to announce the presence of illness or imminence of death. In Bichat's researches lay the origins of what historians of medicine variously refer to as "localism" or "solidism." For only when diseases were "no longer general humoral events," as Ackerknecht well puts it, "but located in different organs, could they be studied and treated separately."[25]

In the localism and solidism of Bichat originated, in turn, that epistemological rupture that would produce a permanent gap or chasm between the older world of Hippocratic or Galenic humoral theory and the new world of anatomico-pathological medicine created by the Paris school. Within several decades, says Jean-Charles Sournia in his recent *Histoire de la médecine*, "disease became something different. It was no longer a subject of discussion, but of material observation."[26] The other important consequence of this epistemological rupture, as we have heard Duffin say, is that it would radically transform the relationship between physician and patient, making disease an entity always potentially visible to the trained professional eye even as it remained unseen by the person in whose body it was harbored. This was the beginning of the conceptual revolution in whose latter stages we live today: what the CAT-scan knows or the MRI knows may well be unknown to me or you, and when we are put in possession of that knowledge it will be by our physician.

The controversy that followed Michel Foucault's *Birth of the Clinic* when it was published in France in 1966 owed not least to the clarity with which it set forth this new and revolutionary element in Paris theory. Historians of medicine tend nowadays to look a bit condescendingly upon *Naissance de la Clinique*, with its emphasis on "the gaze" (*le regard*) and its tendency to reduce the complexities of medical epistemology to mere relations of social domination. Foucault's study nonetheless captures the sense of epistemological rupture, of a new conceptual world coming into existence while an older one was fading into incomprehensibility, that actually did follow from the discoveries of such men as Bichat and Laennec and Pierre Charles Alexandre Louis. The essence of the new clinical gaze, Foucault famously said, lay in its "paradoxical ability to hear a language as soon as it perceives a spectacle."[27] Or in the idea, as he says elsewhere, that "the body must be subjected to a medical examination which will allow it to confess its pathological secrets to the physician, even while concealing them from the patient."[28]

One great value of Oliver Wendell Holmes's medical writings is their acute sense of the epistemological rupture signaled by Paris medicine, which was for him put into perspective by a lifelong fascination with the history of medicine from the days of Hippocrates onwards. Thus it is, for instance, that Holmes would see so clearly that Harvey's *De motu cordis*, considered by many of his contemporaries an isolated curiosity of medical discovery, had in reality been invisibly laying the groundwork for the Parisian discovery of an interior world of the body: "I have heard a very

Oliver Wendell Holmes in Paris

wise physician question whether any important result had accrued to practical medicine from Harvey's discovery of the circulation," remarks Holmes. But pathological anatomy as perfected by the Paris school, undertaken in the same spirit as Harvey's studies, shows the value of pure research: "You have only to read Cullen's description of inflammation of the lungs or of the bowels, and compare it with such as you may find in Laennec or Watson, to see the immense gain which diagnosis and prognosis have derived from general anatomy."[29]

Harvey's discovery of the circulation, in short, lay at the beginning of the movement that has made it possible to conceive of the body as a self-contained physical system obeying its own laws. In a certain sense, this sudden illumination would have retained its revolutionary implications even if the theory of the circulation had for whatever strange reason had no therapeutic consequences at all. Harvey, moreover, had used the new quantitative methods of Baconian science to substantiate his theory, showing, for instance, that only the hypothesis of a relatively small volume of fluid endlessly circulating could be squared with the amount of blood actually contained within the body. He had explained the function of the valves by analogy with the valves used in hydraulic apparatus, permitting a conception of the heart as a pump. And, as important as anything else, he had made the heart as an organ the center of a physical system in which the other organs could be imagined as having similarly vital roles. All this lies in the immediate background of what Holmes means by saying, in the essay just cited, that "Anatomy, Physiology, and Pathology have received a new light" from the anatomico-pathological "method of contemplating the living structures."

In standard histories of medicine, it is usually Morgagni's *De sedibus*, coming over a century after Harvey's work on the circulation, that marks the next stage in the development of physiological theory. Morgagni's contribution is, in fact, unassailable. His great work, based on a lifetime of post mortem dissection and careful analysis of symptoms, is a clear precursor of the Parisian anatomico-pathological view of the body as an interior world in which the lesions discovered in autopsy correspond to the symptoms shown by the patient when alive. At the time Morgagni carried out his researches, his ability to "see into" the body of his patients could seem to physicians trained in the older Galenic theory to be something very nearly approaching magic. Here, for instance, is Morgagni's ante-mortem prediction of the hepatized ("liverlike") lung tissue found in severe cases of pneumonia:

In a convent a nun "was seized, in the night, with a fever, with which she first shivered, and was cold . . . and after that grew hot." Then she showed pain in the side, difficulty in breathing, dry cough, a hard pulse, sense of weight in the thorax. After her death, Morgagni said, "Come, let the body be dissected; this will be certainly found to be the nature of the disease, that the lungs shall appear to have the substance of liver." At the autopsy, he "saw that . . . when they were cut into they appeared to have a dense and compact substance, like that of the liver, as I had predicted." And he continued describing the pneumonia in considerable and excellent detail.[30]

Nonetheless, Morgagni's correlation of external symptoms with internal lesions is one of those conceptual breakthroughs whose originality springs into view only when looked at through the lens of later discoveries. For *De sedibus* was written in a period when the older Galenic or humoral theory still placed a conceptual blockage in the way of any theory based on pathological anatomy, always insisting that illness was unintelligible except as a set of symptoms immediately experienced by the patient. An idea of disease as something working silently away in the interior world of a body outwardly in a state of robust health was, to a physician trained in Galenic medicine, a contradiction in terms. "Many doctors were interested in pathological anatomy," writes Duffin in her *History of Medicine*, thinking not only of Morgagni but of Matthew Baillie's great 1793 work on morbid anatomy, "but they were baffled by its relevance to diagnosis and therapeutics, since both were predicated on symptoms. . . . To have a 'disease' in the eighteenth century, a person had to feel sick."[31]

In his later medical writings, Holmes is always properly respectful of Morgagni's originality as a pathologist, but for him the epistemological revolution associated with Paris medicine had began with the work of Marie-François-Xavier Bichat, the brilliant young researcher whose *Traité des membranes* (1801) Holmes took to have marked an epoch in anatomical and physiological study. For although Bichat would die in 1802 at the age of only thirty-one, he was during his short career a tireless worker, reported to have performed 600 autopsies in the last winter before his death. His *Anatomie générale* would be taken by subsequent generations of Paris medical students as a clarion call to the new anatomico-pathological basis of medical theory: "What is the value of observation," Bichat wrote, "if one does not know the seat of the disease? You can take notes for twenty years from morning to evening at the sickbed on the diseases of the heart, lung, and stomach, and you will reap nothing but confusion. The symptoms, corresponding to nothing, will offer but incoherent phenomena."[32]

As early as the later nineteenth century, French medical historians would be claiming Bichat's work as having inaugurated what Jules Rochard, in his *Histoire de la chirurgie française au XIXe siècle* (1875), was already able to call a "revolution in science." "Two and one-half years," says Rochard, "sufficed for him to produce his prodigious work"; when it was completed, the Bichatian revolution had "constituted science on new bases."[33] For Holmes, this would always remain the essential truth about Bichat's *Anatomie générale*, whose perspective would inform not only his own teaching as a professor of anatomy but his subsequent medical writings. Bichat's real discovery was the interior world of the body. "What geology has done for our knowledge of the earth," Holmes would say, "has been done for the knowledge of the body" by general anatomy: "It is the geology of the body." The revolution in medical thinking is due, he adds, to "the extraordinary genius of Bichat, to whom more than any other we owe this new method of study."[34]

The underlying basis of the Paris medical revolution, Jacalyn Duffin has said, meaning something very close to what Holmes calls the geology of the body, was "the anchoring of diseases to three-dimensional anatomical forms."[35] For American students, it was the way Paris medical teaching permitted them to understand the new relation between external symptoms and internal lesions through frequent and systematic dissection that made this conceptual relation real. For in the United States, as in England, the taboo against dissection of dead bodies had driven generations of medical students to grave robbing—the famous business of the "resurrection men" whose trade would come to sensational light in the trial of Burke and Hare in Edinburgh in 1828—to provide anatomical material. Anatomy riots, so called, were a regular feature of institutional life at American medical schools. "Some foolish and rash fellow," wrote Professor Nathan Smith of Yale Medical School to a friend in the early nineteenth century, "went to West Haven about 20 miles from this place and took a female subject from the ground. . . . This raised a mob who broke more than 100 panes of glass in the building before they could be dispersed."[36]

John Harley Warner has argued that it was the ready availability of bodies for dissection—and not, as he says, the "intellectual vigor" of Paris medicine[37]—that drew vast numbers of foreign students to the École de Médecine. The point has a great deal of plausibility. Consider the experience of John Collins Warren, father of Mason, whose own father had been professor of anatomy at Harvard before him. As a medical student in the 1790s, he and some fellow students dig up of the body of "a stout young man," in the middle of the night, only then realizing that a stranger is standing in the shadows smoking and watching them. Thinking quickly, one of the party goes out a side gate, pretending to be drunk, and distracts the stranger. "The body was then quickly taken up, and packed in the chaise between two of the parties, who drove off to Cambridge with their booty. Two of us stayed to fill the grave: but my companions, being alarmed, soon left the burying-ground. . . . I got off without further interruption; drove, with the tools, to Cambridge, and arrived there just before daylight. When my father . . . found I had been engaged in this scrape, he was very much alarmed; but when the body was uncovered, and he saw what a fine healthy subject it was, he seemed to be as much pleased as I ever saw him. This body lasted the course through."[38]

In Paris, by comparison, students discovered a paradise for anatomical study. At the Clamart and the École Pratique d'Anatomie, we recall Augustus Gardner saying, conveniently situated at the center of the Latin Quarter, four thousand bodies are provided annually for dissection: "Every day, at twelve o'clock, there is a distribution of them among all classes of students." In addition, instructors in anatomy have each a small building for the use of themselves and their students, each with ten or fifteen tables of cast iron: "The human body may thus be viewed in every stage of dissection."[39] One of the most vivid accounts of this sector of Paris medicine is given by Holmes in a letter written home to his parents in 1835. He is describing dissection at the Clamart:

> This establishment is not one of the little infernal suffocating holes in which the unhappy native of our uncivilized land is often obliged to pursue his labors, but a spacious courtyard with several neat white halls, and a garden and fountain in the middle. In these precincts hundreds of students dissect during a part of the year and operate during another. After having taken our lessons in operative surgery, a Swiss friend of mine—whose intimacy has been enjoyed successively by poor Jackson, by Bowditch, and now by myself,—the Swiss student and myself, I say, bought a few cheap instruments together, and began to make ourselves operators. It is an odd thing for anybody but a medical student to think of, that human flesh should be sold like beef or mutton. But at twelve o'clock every day, the hour of distribution of subjects, you might have seen M. Bizot and myself—like the old gentlemen one sometimes sees at a market—choosing our day's provision with the same epicurean nicety. We paid fifty sous apiece for our subject, and before evening we had cut him into inch pieces. Now all this can hardly be done anywhere in the world but at Paris. . . .[40]

Yet Mason Warren, as the son of a Harvard professor of anatomy, was one of the very few American students who did not need to travel to Paris or spend hours at the Clamart to train himself in anatomical study, for he had long been permitted to assist at the autopsies his father regularly performed on fatal cases. When Mason departed for Paris in 1832, he carried with him an extraordinary document entitled "Rules for the daily conduct of life and for professional progress," composed by his father to guide his son's studies at the École de Médicine. His son, says John Collins Warren, is to direct his attention to the practice of surgery. ("Observe operations. Get as near as possible. Anticipate the steps.") He is, specifically, not to waste his time on dissection: "*Anatomical dissection not to be pursued abroad. It can be done at home, and would occupy too much time*" (my italics). Among the operations he is to observe are those for lithotomy and, in particular, lithotrity as performed by M. Civiale: "observe his instruments."[41]

This, as we have seen, was a paternal injunction that Mason obeyed at the earliest opportunity, visiting Civiale in October, 1832. Some ten months later he would again watch Civiale perform a lithotrity, this time after having observed numerous standard lithotomies, what both surgeons and patients more normally called "cutting for the stone," performed by the great Dupuytren and such lesser surgeons as Sanson and Roux. To compare Mason's first and second accounts of Civiale is to get some sense of why Valentine Mott was moved to virtual rhapsody—"How much pain," we remember Mott exclaiming, "how much agony, has not this great and good man saved to his fellow-creatures!"—in describing Civiale's procedure. Here is Mason's second report:

> The operator standing on the right side of the patient, seizes the penis with the left hand and with the right introduces the instrument properly oiled . . . into the urethra. In passing it into the bladder hardly the slightest degree of force is employed, the instrument being allowed first to slip slowly by its own force perpendicularly to the curve in the urethra. . . . In this part of the operation Civiale is unique. . . . When the stone is discovered to be well within the grip of the instrument, a handle is affixed to its free extremities and being given to an assistant the stone is ground by turning the *paret* swiftly round with a bow made for the purpose. . . . The pain suffered by the patient during the operation is . . . hardly to be mentioned and its after effects are usually a slight febrile attack. . . .[42]

The sense of barely-suppressed wonder evident in Mason's latest account, what Valentine Mott had in mind in speaking of "the delicacy of tact and adroitness of execution" displayed by Civiale, or in saying that "it is utterly impossible for any one to imagine the highly finished style of his manipulations," arises from his sense that he is witnessing a scene in which that interior world of the body brought into visibility by Paris medicine has been made available to surgeons as well as pathologists. Mason is witnessing, in short, the Parisian triumph of what would variously be called regional or surgical anatomy, which his friend Oliver Wendell Holmes would some years later also compare to geology in the study of the earth. The new surgical anatomy, Holmes would say, enables the surgeon "to see with the mind's eye through the opaque tissues down to the bone on which they lie, as if the skin were transparent as the cornea, and the organs it covers as the gelatinous pulp of a medusa."[43]

Civiale's procedure was a triumph of the new "geology of the body" as it had been born in relation to another element in the radical reorganization of the Paris hospital system. This was the equalizing of surgery and medicine in medical training. For surgeons prior to the Revolution, as Jacalyn Duffin says, were "often illiterate and traditionally inferior to physicians," in guild terms belonging not to medicine but to "the barber class, who derived income from shaving, cutting hair, and drawing teeth."[44] Ambroise Paré, for instance, one of the greatest figures in the history of surgery, had in the late 16th century learned his trade by apprenticeship to a barber. The most important innovation in Paris medical teaching, L. W. B. Brockliss has argued, really came in 1803, when "it was decided to join together under one institutional umbrella the formation of physicians and surgeons," something that medical reformers had insistently been calling for "on the grounds that the two professions were so mutually dependent that their traditional separation was ridiculous."[45]

Nothing illustrates more dramatically than Civiale's operation the way the Paris medical revolution had brought into visibility for physicians and surgeons alike an interior world of the body never before glimpsed in medical theory. For when Mason watched the standard operations for bladder stone performed by surgeons like Dupuytren and Roux, he was watching variations on a procedure that goes back to the beginnings of recorded history. The earliest bladder stone known to us, found by archaeologists in Egypt, was formed in the body of its owner sometime around 4300 B.C. In ancient Greece, the stone, in medical terminology called a vesicle calculus, was so common that Hippocrates felt it necessary to warn his own students about the dangers of the operation to remove it. "To cut through the bladder is lethal," goes one section of the Hippocratic oath. "I will not cut for stone. I will leave this operation to be performed by practitioners"—by which he meant the itinerant stonecutters who could still be found wandering the European countryside as late as the end of the eighteenth century.

For a number of reasons, probably having to do largely with changes in diet, the bladder stone has in our own time become a curiosity of medical history, but for thousands of years it was a major source of physical agony for vast numbers of suffering men and women. To observe the stones that survive today in medical museums—a specimen on display in the Hunterian Museum in London, for instance, weighs 44 ounces and measures 16 inches in circumference—is to get some idea of what sufferers went through. Readers of Pepys's *Diary* will remember the terrible pain that would finally drive him, knowing full well that its extraction involved an operation scarcely less dangerous than the condition itself, into the hands of a London surgeon. For years afterwards, wholly aware that his having survived was very nearly a medical miracle, he would hold a celebration on the anniversary of his operation, and subsequently would have the stone mounted in a box for his own contemplation and display to friends.

The stone was particularly dangerous for males, for whom the urethra, the long membranous tube running through the center of the penis into the bladder, prevented the easier voiding of the calculus often permitted to women, and in whom the prostate, situated at just the point at which the surgeon would otherwise wish to cut through into the bladder, presented a surgical obstacle that had to be circumvented. The oldest operation for the stone was through a simple perineal incision, the perineum being the anatomical area lying between the scrotal sac and the anus. The itinerant stone-cutter of the ancient or medieval world, with a knowledge of regional anatomy passed down within the trade, was able to insert a finger into the rectum and press down on the stone from above, slice through the neck of the bladder ahead of the prostate, and extract the calculus either with his fingers or, in later centuries, with a specially-designed forceps. The incision was then normally left open for the drainage of urine.

It was, observes Harold Ellis in his *History of the Bladder Stone*, "only the terrible and protracted agonies produced by the stone that gave men sufficient courage to place themselves under the lithotomist's cruel instruments."[46] The pain of the operation was so agonizing that the great problem for the surgeon was keeping the patient still enough to carry out a delicate set of procedures. The standard solution was to bind the patient in what was known as the lithotomy position—the term is still used in connection with childbirth—and have him held down by assistants. In 1575, the great French surgeon Ambroise Paré gave precise directions: "The patient shall be placed upon a firm table or bench with . . . a pillow under his loins and back, so that he may lie half upright with his thighs lifted up and his legs and heels drawn back to his buttocks. Then shall his feet be bound with a ligature of three fingers breadth passed about his ankles, and . . . both his hands shall be bound to his knees. The patient thus bound, it is fit you have four strong men at hand; that is, two to hold his arms, and the other two who may so firmly and straitly hold the knee with one hand, and the foot with the other, that he may neither move his limbs nor stir his buttocks but be forced to keep the same posture with his whole body."[47]

Even with the new and more precise knowledge of surgical anatomy given to the Parisian surgeon, the operation was hardly relieved of its terrors for both doctor and patient. Consider, for instance, an operation for the stone described by C. B. Tilanus, a Dutch physician who had gone to Paris to complete his surgical training and would later become Professor of Surgery at the University of Amsterdam. The protagonist of the story is Dupuytren, at this point some thirteen years younger than when Mason Warren would watch him perform the same operation:

> January 13, 1819. Hôtel Dieu. A man of thirty-eight has suffered since he was a boy of six or seven from difficult and painful micturition. This became accompanied by pain in the kidneys and vomiting, and he soon began to pass small stones. His manual occupation caused these pains to increase, so that now they are unbearable. He has never been seriously examined and came to find relief. Dupuytren found a stone on his first sounding. It is probably of considerable size, having been in existence twenty-five or twenty-six years; moreover, it can be felt above the pubis and far into the rectum, and with a hand on the pubis and a finger in the rectum the stone can be felt by both and its size to some extent determined. The patient begs to be operated on on account of the terrible pain. The pain in the kidneys, which has been present so many years, is an important contra-indication. They fear that three or four days after the operation there is sure to be inflammation in the diseased kidneys, and then fever and death. They also fear they may find a diseased bladder. A small amount of urine is examined and found to contain small quantities of mucus and pus.

For Dupuytren, the size of the stone presents an all but insurmountable problem. The calculus is much too large to be extracted through a perineal incision, the operation at which Dupytren is an acknowledged master. His alternative is then the suprapubic incision, called the "high operation," that had been given currency by the most famous of the itinerant stone-cutters, one Frère Côme. Using a set of instruments called the *apparatus altus,* this consisted of slicing into the bladder above the pubic bone, which in addition to cutting through the abdominal muscles ran a great risk of damaging the peritoneum, the membranous sac that surrounds most of the abdominal and pelvic region and holds the intestines in place. One of Bichat's most important discoveries had been that any injury to this tissue was overwhelmingly likely to result in peritonitis, a rapidly-spreading inflammation of the membrane almost always fatal to the patient. In addition, there was great danger of inflammation and infection by dispersion of urine into the surgical wound.

There is one other possibility. This patient has a stone so large that it is bulging perceptibly through the wall of the rectum. In theory, it ought to be possible to go into the bladder through the rectum, slicing through the sphincter and extracting the stone through an incision in the intestinal wall. Though the operation has never been tried—there is an obvious danger of infiltration of the wound by feces—the peculiarities of this case justify at least entertaining the idea. The way Dupuytren goes about testing the possibility is a virtual parable of Paris surgical anatomy during this period. Having inserted a large stone by internal incision into the bladder of a corpse, he tries the rectal operation as it would have to be performed on a living patient. On his first attempt, he extracts the stone with enormous difficulty. In trials on two subsequent corpses, he convinces himself that, even if he were able to remove the stone in this way, the surgical trauma would be too great to give the patient any chance of survival. "Nothing remains therefore," reports Tilanus in his diary, "but the *apparatus altus*. It will take place tomorrow."[48]

The next day, Dupuytren performs the operation using Frère Côme's method. The incision is three to four inches long. The abdominal muscles are severed on the diagonal to prevent their contraction from interfering with the procedure. After some struggle, Dupuytren extracts a stone 3½ inches long, with a smooth side showing that it has been rubbing against another stone. The second stone, as large as the first, is extracted, a small incision is made through the perineum and a catheter inserted to drain urine from the bladder, and the patient is bandaged. "The patient," reports Tilanus, "is put to bed with chest up, knees drawn so as not to strain the abdominal muscles. A venesection in an hour's time and strict diet is prescribed to avoid severe inflammation. The venesection to be repeated if the pain becomes severe."[49] The outcome is a sad illustration of the terrible risks involved in surgery before asepsis and antibiotics:

January 19, Hôtel Dieu. The patient died. An hour after the operation there was difficulty in breathing, three 'palettes' of blood were taken. During the day he was peaceful; urine was evacuated by the cannula . . . and soothing drinks were given him. In the evening he had two applications of twenty-five leeches each in the region of the kidneys. The night was peaceful too. Sunday morning he felt well; his eyes were clear, his breathing full and his abdomen soft. He complained of a gnawing pain in his stomach, which he ascribed to hunger, and begged for food; a few spoonfuls of broth were given him; the pulse was frequent. Towards noon feverish shiverings; the abdomen becomes painful, his appearance bad, his breathing difficult, his pulse very frequent, twenty-five leeches are placed on the abdomen. At the evening visit he already appeared moribund; a palette of blood was drawn with the order that it should be repeated every three hours. This, however, was not necessary, for at eleven he died.[50]

In an age innocent of germ theory, the great danger lay in postoperative infection. The agent of this patient's death was probably what in Dupuytren's day was called erysipelas, which we now recognize as streptococcus pyogenes, so common in surgery that, in combination with the anaerobes that then invaded the badly compromised tissue, it came to be called hospital gangrene. The cause of death was almost undoubtedly septic shock, a cascade reaction to toxicity that even today is not entirely understood. "The entire evolving syndrome," explains Sherwin Nuland, "is thought to represent an inflammatory response to the presence in the blood of microbial and other invaders that generate toxic substances. . . . The lung and other organs seem to create and release certain chemical substances that have a deleterious effect on blood vessels, organs, and even cells, including the elements of the blood. The tissue cells become incapable of extracting sufficient oxygen from hemoglobin at about the same time that less hemoglobin is being brought to them by the reduced circulation. These events so much resemble the classical picture of cardiogenic or hypovolemic shock that their total effect is called septic shock." Today, it is possible to try to combat the condition with antibiotics and other measures, though these are often unsuccessful. In Dupuytren's time, the result was a foregone conclusion: "the vital organs fail one after the other."[51]

This is the agony from which Civiale's operation of lithotrity had saved hundreds of patients, the reason that Valentine Mott is moved to speak in terms of awe and wonder at what today seems little more than a rudimentary procedure. Mott can scarcely be accused of exaggerating in calling Civiale "one of the noblemen of our profession," a "great and good man" who has saved his fellow creatures an endless amount of pain and agony. For Civiale's patients all survived, having undergone little more than the slight discomfort involved in the original insertion of the *lithotome* into the bladder, some asking Civiale, when he had already crushed the stone into fragments, when the operation would begin. It is what Mott calls the delicacy and tact of Civiale's procedure—he is thinking of the Latin *tactus*, the term for the surgeon's delicate touch—that Mason will endlessly practice in the evenings when he has returned to his Paris lodgings. "The rules with regard to the difference of the operation on the living urethra exposed to its spasmodic action," he writes his father in 1835, "I cannot at present resolve. I keep a very nice instrument of the last and most simple improvement at my room and exercise daily on ox and hog bladders."[52]

Dupuytren's order to bleed the patient after the operation brings into view the one major area in which the anatomico-pathological conception of disease had not conquered the older humoral theory. For the concept of "plethora" had dictated bloodletting for over two thousand years, and in the new Paris setting had simply been reformulated as a remedy against inflammation, under the new and scientific-sounding name of "antiphlogistic" treatment. Yet the measures taken by Dupuytren would have been instantly recognizable to physicians a hundred years earlier. "No operation of surgery is so frequently necessary as bleeding," wrote William Buchan in *Domestic Medicine*, the famous eighteenth-century guide to home medical care. "Bleeding is proper at the beginning of all inflammatory fevers, as pleurisies, peripneumonies, etc. It is likewise proper in all topical inflammations, as those of the intestines, womb, bladder, stomach, kidneys, throat, eyes, etc. as also in the asthma, sciatic pains, coughs, head-aches, rheumatisms."[53]

The amount of blood proper to be taken was, as Dupuyten's orders about his patient suggest, considerable. The "palette" mentioned by Tilanus was a clinical measure equal to four ounces. Another patient mentioned by Tilanus suggests how routine this was: "The girl with the broken forearm is in danger. The inflammation in the chest continues, notwithstanding four blood-lettings and four applications of leeches. This has made her very weak."[54] In a letter to his father, Mason Warren described a case in which the patient clearly succumbed not to the operation—a procedure on a 23-year-old man meant merely to remove a foreign body from the knee joint—but to the post-operative treatment:

> Lisfranc operated making an incision over the body. . . . After extraction the body was severed without difficulty. . . . The knee was ordered to be kept perfectly still; patient to be bled to 16 oz. and 40 leeches applied. The next morning the patient having been somewhat restless in the night . . . bleeding was ordered of 16 oz. and 80 leeches to the knee. The third day bleeding of 8 oz.; 4th of 4. Blood-letting was then discontinued on account of the feebleness of patient . . . . [for a month after operation] abscesses of increased size continued to form exteriously to the joint and the patient died on the 27th worn out by the diarrhea which he had been troubled with the last 16 or 17 days of his life.[55]

In conceptual terms, the older humoral notion of bloodletting as a treatment for inflammation, consorting as oddly as it did with the new anatomico-pathological view of disease as arising from internal lesions, led to an impasse in medical theory. When Oliver Wendell Holmes arrives in Paris the next year, he will attend a course on internal pathology in which the brilliant young physician Gabriel Andral will dwell in great detail on all the diseases that cannot be explained in terms of local lesions. "Open a few corpses," we recall Bichat saying, and the obscurity surrounding the patient's external symptoms will disappear. But opening a few corpses does nothing to explain the etiology of so common a disease as malaria, in that day known as "intermittent fever," or the great multitude of diseases that we should today recognize as being due to microbial invaders or endocrine disorders. For all his awareness of an important debt to the Bichatian revolution in tissue pathology, Andral will be simultaneously aware that the new localism and solidism of the Paris school have left a great deal to be explained by medical research.

In practical terms, on the other hand, the growing gap between such humoral remedies as venesection and the discoveries of the new anatomico-pathological medicine would produce a therapeutic hiatus, a significant period during which medical theory has outstripped therapeutics, and during which the emphasis of enlightened physicians has shifted towards what in Paris medicine was known as the *méthode expectante*, or doing nothing harmful to the patient while doing one's best to aid the body's natural powers of recovery. Literally translated as the "expectant method," this approach to therapy would become the virtual badge of Paris-trained physicians in the United States in the mid-nineteenth century. One of Holmes's companions on his voyage across the Atlantic, Dr. Jacob Bigelow, would provide its manifesto in his famous essay on "Self-Limited Diseases." For Holmes himself, as we shall see, it would have profound implications for the metaphysics underwriting *The Autocrat of the Breakfast Table* and the later volumes of the Breakfast Table trilogy.

For American students, the brilliant achievements of the anatomico-pathological school and justification for the *méthode expectante* converged in the teaching of Pierre Charles Alexandre Louis, whose painstaking studies in tissue pathology produced results that could then be extrapolated through the "numerical system" that was his own greatest contribution to Paris medicine. Mason Warren captures something of the impact made by Louis as an apostle of the new interior world of the body discovered by Paris medicine: "in the autopsies made by Louis he examines every organ no matter what the disease may be, the Brain, Lungs and Larynx, Heart, all the different abdominal organs, the Intestines cut open from one end to the other and all the morbid appearances described, the mesenteric glands, the aorta, etc. By going thus thoroughly through with his examination Louis has been able to throw great light on many diseases whose pathology has been hitherto unknown and of course [destroy many] of the absurd doctrines that have crept into medicine."[56]

During the course of the same researches, Louis had also unexpectedly discovered that many of the therapeutic measures drawn from the older Galenic or humoral medicine, and especially the practice of copious bloodletting, were not only useless but actually dangerous to patients. "What Louis did was this," recalled Holmes in his last address to his Harvard class. "He showed by a strict analysis of numerous cases that bleeding did not strangle,—*jugulate* was the word then used,—acute diseases, more especially pneumonia. This was not a reform,—it was a revolution."[57] It is directly from the bedside rounds of Louis at La Pitié that American students like James Jackson, Jr., Mason Warren, and Holmes himself would carry back to their own country the disturbing news that doctors who blindly followed the protocols of the old Galenic regimen were not only doing nothing to cure their patients, but were very often killing them. As we shall see, Holmes's lifelong allegiance to the *méthode expectante*, involving the notion of a *vis medicatrix naturae* or "healing power of nature" in which he would come to see important theological implications, had its origins in these same daily rounds at La Pitié.

A reader of Mason Warren's letters to his father can sense the nearly irresistible gravitational pull, all during his two years in Paris, of the new conception of disease associated with Louis's pathological researches. Mason had been sent to Paris to learn advanced surgical technique. He has been assiduous in his attendance on the lectures and demonstrations of such men as Dupuytren and Lisfranc and Roux. As the stipulated period of his Paris stay draws to a close, then, it comes as little surprise to find Mason writing home to ask for another year of study in Paris, this time with Louis, "the greatest pathologist in the world at the present day": "His manner of examining disease and his philosophical way of teaching has a most wonderful effect in showing exactly what and how little we know of internal pathology and points out the only true way of arriving at satisfactory results, this by numbering cases. The effect which following Louis properly has had on the minds of those of my acquaintances who have been with him is such as would alone determine me to make great sacrifices to spend 5 or 6 months with him."[58]

In writing to his father, Mason was careful to stress that he was in no way thinking about deserting surgery for internal medicine. One of the main points of his spending additional time in Paris to study with Louis was precisely, he was careful to add, that "I think the principles which he establishes with regard to medicine can be carried with great advantage into the study of surgery."[59] This is the basis on which John Collins Warren would accede to the proposal. "You will be expected, he wrote to Mason from Boston on August 22, 1834, "to come home with a perfect knowledge of the manual of surgical operations in the most improved form. You will be expected to be fully acquainted with auscultation and percussion . . . and to be well acquainted with the prevalent medical doctrines. A deficiency in these points would not fail to be noticed. For the rest, besides possessing a reasonable knowledge of the healing art, you ought to bring home, if possible, something new and striking, at the same time guarding your acquirements with the respect for others without which a medical man cannot be liked by his profession."[60]

Among the new and striking accomplishments that Mason Warren would bring home from Paris would be Civiale's operation for lithotrity, to which he would introduce his father when he joined him in medical practice. He was an early pioneer in modern plastic surgery, reintroducing an operation for rhinoplasty—reconstruction of the nose using a live skin graft from the patient's arm—that had been pioneered by Indian surgeons centuries before but never practiced with consistent success in the United States. In October 1846, at Massachusetts General Hospital, he would assist John Collins Warren in the first surgical operation performed under ether. Shortly thereafter, he would perform the first private operation in which the patient was anesthetized under ether, and in the same year would become the first surgeon to use anesthesia when operating on a child. For thirty-two years, despite the chronic ill health from which he had suffered since his Harvard undergraduate days, Mason would occupy a prominent place in the Massachusetts medical profession, before succumbing to a wasting illness in 1867, at the age of fifty-six.

Upon Mason's return from Paris in 1835, he was immediately able to take over part of the burden of his father's medical practice, winning the confidence both of his father's patients and other senior Boston physicians called in to consult on difficult cases. His impact on these older physicians was no doubt partly due to the glamour of the new Paris medicine to which he had devoted so much assiduous study, but it was due as well to personal qualities that impressed all with whom he came in contact. So immediately successful was Mason that in the summer after his return his father, whose profession had up to then consumed virtually every moment of his time, was able to turn over his practice to his son and take a protracted vacation in the Southern states. Two years later, John Collins Warren would be able to turn his practice entirely over to Mason and depart for Paris to himself follow the famous hospital teachers whose lectures and demonstrations his son had been attending just a short time before.

There is something strangely moving in this picture of a Harvard medical professor, already at the very height of his profession in the United States, taking his anonymous place among the crowd of medical students surrounding Louis, now moved from La Pitié to the Hôtel Dieu, as he makes his clinical rounds. "When I approached the bed where he was making his visit with the aid of a dimly burning candle, towering in the midst of his pupils," reported Warren in a letter written from Paris in 1837, "I saw a tall, upright man, with a countenance rather pale, bearing the marks of sagacity and deep reflection. He was intently occupied with his patient, and seemed to be conscious of nothing but what was related to him. His inquiries were very minute; and, when the patient gave him doubtful answers (which he frequently did), he repeated the questions. . . . He then gave to the students a brief abstract of the history of the case, his opinion as to its nature, and terminated with a prescription."[61]

From this visit to Paris, John Collins Warren would return to become the surgeon always remembered for performing the first operation under anesthesia, a leader of the medical profession in the United States, and a teacher of anatomy and physiology from whom generations of Harvard medical students learned the rudiments of their profession. When he died in 1856, another Harvard professor of anatomy would contribute a graceful eulogy to the man who had so dominated Massachusetts medicine for nearly half a century. In the last years of Warren's life, said this eulogist, the aging physician had found a just reward for his strenuous years of toil: "he had got out of the brawling current," and was able to devote himself to his favorite studies in the new science of paleontology, studying the fossil remains in which "the life of the eternity that is past has left its earliest autographs": "he pursued his cheerful labors to the last, bent, but not broken, and so walked softly from among us into the land of shadows."[62] The eulogy was pronounced by John Collins Warren's successor as professor of anatomy at Harvard, a younger man who, at the moment Mason Warren was already in Paris observing Civiale perform a lithotrity, was still at home in Cambridge, just making up his mind to abandon the study of law in favor of medicine—Dr. Oliver Wendell Holmes.

CHAPTER TWO

The School of La Charité

A letter from Holmes to his parents in early November, 1833, just over six months after his arrival in Paris, captures the excitement that swept through newly-arrived medical students as the winter course of lectures got underway: "The whole walls round the Ecole de Médecine are covered with notices of lectures, the greater part of them gratuitous; the dissecting-rooms, which accommodate six hundred students, are open; the lessons are ringing aloud through all the great hospitals. The students from all lands are gathered together, and the great harvest of the year is open to us."[1] The same note may be heard in scores of letters written by foreign medical students in Paris in the 1820s and 1830s, a sense of wonder not only that such shining opportunity exists in a single city, but that it is free to all who come. In Paris, wrote Augustus Gardner, the portals of institutions of learning "are thrown wide open, and the rich and poor stand on equal ground. Lectures are daily delivered on every subject, with which man is conversant, by professors of the profoundest learning. . . . No wonder the Frenchman feels so keenly the *amour de patrie.*"[2]

Holmes had landed at Havre in early May. Under the expert guidance of his Boston friends Mason Warren, Henry Bowditch, and James Jackson, Jr., all of whom were already students in the Paris hospitals, he had immediately gotten his bearings in the otherwise perplexing world that greeted foreign medical students. It was, as another American medical visitor reported, a world that did not stretch much beyond the limits of the ancient Latin Quarter, home of the École de Médecine and the major hospitals, "where all the medical students and many of the professors, private lecturers, demonstrators, medical-book sellers, instrument makers, medical artistes, anatomical workers in wax and papier-maché, preparers of natural and artificial skeletons, and other varieties of surgical and anatomical specimens reside; where the streets are so narrow and filthy, and without pavements or sidewalks, as to endanger life at every corner."[3] The topography of *Paris médicale*, as it was called in a guidebook widely used by foreign students a few years later, extended from the Île de la Cité, where the great Hôtel Dieu rose alongside the cathedral of Notre Dame, to the Jardin des Plantes and the Salpêtrière, about two miles to the east.[4]

This would be Holmes's world for the next two years. He fell easily and at once into the routine followed by his Boston friends, rising early in the morning to attend hospital rounds and clinical lectures, doing dissections at the Clamart in the afternoon, and at a somewhat later period making time to observe the procedures developed by famous surgeons like Velpeau and Roux. "Roux," he would recall for an audience of Boston physicians some years later, "is a robust, square, grey headed man of exceeding quickness in his speech and all his movements. He is essentially an operating surgeon—carnivorous, anthrophagous by nature."[5] A sense of Roux's intrepidity can be gotten from Mason Warren's Paris letters:

> Roux attempted the extirpation of an immense tumeur of the neck extending from the parotid to the clavicle and from the thyroid gland before to the middle of the neck behind. Roux had flattered himself that the tumeur was either encysted or had some determined boundaries in the cellular membrane. After however two incisions over the tumeur and a very long and tedious dissection with ligature to the carotid and jugular vein which last overflowed the operator with blood, the tumeur was found to be cancerous with the larger artery and veins passing directly through its centre and the operation relinquished as offering no possible hopes of success.[6]

Although Holmes felt the pull of both surgery and medicine—in 1839, shortly after he assumed the professorship of anatomy at Dartmouth Medical School,[7] the University of Maryland would offer him its chair in surgery—the enthusiasm of his friends James Jackson, Jr. and Henry Bowditch drew him inexorably into the orbit of Pierre Charles Alexandre Louis, the great internal pathologist of the hospital of La Pitié, and so into an emphasis on bedside or clinical teaching. In practice, this meant immediate attendance on Louis's morning rounds at La Pitié, and subsequently, when winter lectures began, the clinic of Auguste Chomel at the Hôtel Dieu and the lectures of Gabriel Andral at the École de Médecine. Though he could hardly have realized the full implications of his choice at the time, Holmes was thus situating himself at the very heart of what one contemporary French medical theorist would call the "school of La Charité,"[8] by which he meant Chomel, Andral, and Louis as standard-bearers of the revolution in diagnostic procedure, and therefore of the new conception of disease as an autonomous entity, that had begun with Laennec's invention of the stethoscope.

By the time he returned home several years later, Holmes would have attended two courses of Chomel's clinical lectures. His notebooks provide a virtual metric of his entry into Paris medicine, from hesitant beginnings to total and confident immersion. Consider, from the first, made up of notes taken shortly after his arrival in 1833, the case of a *couturière*, age 24, who has come to the Hôtel Dieu complaining of stomach pains: "10 days since pain in hypogastric region with frequent desire to pass urine. . . . Kept bed—pain increased. A second pain began in r.[ight] hypoch.[ondrium]. Vomiting of yellow bitter fluid. Since debut headache thirst inappetance [Fr: lack of appetite]—not able to quit bed from pain in abd.[omen]."[9] Then, a year and a half later, in the spring of 1835: "Cas de douleur suivant la bord exterieur du tibia—Il parait douteux à M. Chomel si cette douleur est rheumatismale ou nerveuse.—Il remarque que dans les affections rheumatismales quelques soit les paries qu'elles attaquent, ordinariement, le rheumatism commence par attaquer les articulations—ou des parties ordinariement le siège de la rheumatisme. . . M. Chomel va appliquer deux vessicatoires une à l'origin et l'autre à le point de termination de la douleur."[10]

The fluent French of Holmes's second set of notes is a useful measure of his nearly effortless adjustment to the world of *Paris médicale*. For most American medical students arriving in Paris, learning the language was a major obstacle. Years later, for instance, Henry Bowditch, who graduated in Mason Warren's class at Harvard Medical School and traveled to Europe with him, would recall that he had been compelled to exile himself from his American friends, taking his meals entirely in the company of French and Swiss students, in order to get his French good enough to follow the lectures of Louis, Chomel, and Andral.[11] The same theme recurs in Mason Warren's letters to his father. An English physician, he reports, has kindly provided him a letter of introduction to Dr. Foville, of Rouen, but "I cannot speak French, and until I do, I shall keep clear of all French physicians to whom I have an introduction."[12] Or, similarly, his very first letter after arrival: "the language I find more difficult than I had expected. For the common questions in regard to the necessaries of life I find it easy to make myself understood, but when it comes to anything with conversation am entirely lost."[13]

Throughout his life, Holmes would demonstrate a extraordinary facility for languages, reading Latin as a living language—the long Latin footnotes in his *Medical Essays* are not there for show, but for the benefit of those who shared his own exuberant delight in reading the old medical writers—and Greek adequately. French was not difficult. "I understand my French lectures almost as perfectly as English,"[14] he wrote his brother shortly after arrival. This was not exaggeration meant to impress a younger sibling. "French is a second mother tongue to me almost," he would write his parents in November 1834. "On many subjects I not infrequently think in it. . . . It is quite pleasant to multiply in this way the medium of solution for one's thoughts—and, to express an idea to yourself with exactness, to be able to make change as it were by means of two different metals."[15] This is the Holmes who, twenty years later, will be able to introduce a piece like "Le Rat des Salons à Lecture" into *The Autocrat of the Breakfast Table*, having a bit of fun with the beginner's tribulations with the French language but doing so in a way that testifies to real literary sophistication in the language.

The problem with Chomel's lectures lay elsewhere. Now at the Hôtel Dieu, Auguste Chomel had a few years earlier succeeded the great R. T. H. Laennec at La Charité, the smaller hospital at which Corvisart, in reviving the art of percussion, and Laennec, in inventing auscultation, or exploration of the interior cavity of the chest with the stethoscope, had revolutionized clinical teaching. Chomel's own method of bedside teaching, he would tell the students who followed him on rounds at La Charité, was of very recent date: "MM Corvisart and Laennec were the first to undertake it."[16] Originally a physician much influenced by Pinel's *Nosographie philosophique*—that Linnaean system of classifications that, as we have heard Ackerknecht say, worked by elevating symptoms to the rank of disease units—he had been converted by his La Charité colleagues into a resourceful clinician who took full advantage of the new methods of percussion and auscultation, and whose teaching always included public autopsies of patients whose cases had had an unsuccessful outcome, in order to explain, as he told his students, "the symptoms we have observed during life by the morbid appearances found after death."[17]

By the time Holmes arrived in Paris, however, Chomel had sometime since moved to the larger and more prestigious Hôtel Dieu, his fame as a clinical teacher having drawn more students than could be accommodated in the more confined surroundings of La Charité. And therein, for many students, lay the problem. For Chomel at La Charité had been the very model of the new Paris clinician as teacher, permitting students to share in the physical examinations, summarizing the results of each day's rounds in a lecture immediately following, and then conducting the *leçon* at which autopsies were performed on previous cases. But by 1833, to the frustration of many American students, Chomel had become one of those luminaries to whom *Paris médicale* once refers as the princes of medicine. "I have made two or three attempts to follow Chomel at Hotel Dieu," reported James Jackson, Jr. to his physician father in the year previous to Holmes's arrival, "—but it is impossible to do so with advantage. . . . The visit at Hotel Dieu is commenced an hour and a half before clear daylight, by candle-light, indeed;—there are from two or three hundred pupils in the wards at the same time, and one is fortunate if he sees four patients, and examines one in the course of the visit."[18]

For young Jackson, as for Henry Bowditch and Mason Warren and the brilliant William Gerhard of Philadelphia, the solution was to attend the clinical rounds of P. C. A. Louis at the smaller and more distant hospital of La Pitié. The consequences for American medicine, as Sir William Osler pointed out in a famous essay, would be profound. For Louis, who had begun his own series of groundbreaking clinical observations as Chomel's protegé at La Charité—he had no official position, and was given access to Chomel's wards simply through collegial generosity—was in the process of developing that "numerical method" that would make so lasting an impression on American teachers and practitioners, and in particular on the Oliver Wendell Holmes who would return from Paris to compose an epochal essay on puerperal fever. We will discuss Louis's enormous impact on this group of young Americans in the next chapter. His importance at the outset, as Holmes was settling into his Paris routine, was that Louis's rounds at La Pitié provided an alternative to the frustrations of trying to follow Chomel at the Hôtel Dieu.

For those who had come to Paris meaning to master the essentials of the new anatomico-pathological view of disease, in short, Chomel's clinical lectures combined with Louis's bedside instruction at La Pitié constituted the best of all possible Parisian medical worlds. "I call it a black day," young James Jackson would report to his father concerning Louis's rounds, "in which I have not examined as many as six patients, at least, who present stethoscopic phenomena." In addition to which, "Louis gives a little clinique at each bed."[19] Under the guidance of James Jackson and Mason Warren, this was the setting into which Holmes was introduced almost immediately upon his settling in at 55 rue M. le Prince. In the notes Holmes took during Louis's bedside rounds, we are still able to hear the voice of the teacher speaking directly to his students. Consider the case of a female domestic servant, age 21, who has come into the hospital with symptoms that suggest a number of serious conditions, including enlargement of the heart, tuberculosis, and perhaps pneumonia. Holmes's notes:

> The flatness in the præcord.[ial] reg.[ion]—and the fremissement cataire confirm the supposition which must be admitted of organic disease of the heart. . . . —Fremissement cataire—considered as a sign of rétrécissement [Fr: shrinkage, contraction] of the valves.—In all the cases of rétrécisse[ment] of the valves which I know there is edema

if there is rétrécisse[ment]. It is not probable that there is in this case a rétrécisse[ment] of the valves, notwithstanding the fremissement cataire.—So much for the heart.

Bronchial resp.[iration] and prolonged exp.[iration] on the right side. Bronchophony.

Importance of the general symptoms in this case. Supposition of pneumonia to account for these signs. . . . The problem cannot be rigorously resolved.—The probability is for a tuberculous affection.

But this is not all. The sound of percussion is clearer on the right side and the resp.[iration] more feeble.—The coincidence of this emphysema does not render more probable a dilatation of the bronch.[ia] as the latter has not been found to be more frequent when the other exists.[20]

Out of Holmes's compressed jottings, the new world of Paris anatomic-pathological diagnosis springs into clear view, only slightly obscured by the diagnostic vocabulary of an earlier day. The great point to be made about that diagnostic vocabulary—bronchophony, the *fremissement cataire*, dullness in the præcordium, all of which we shall discuss shortly—is that it is new and radical, a direct consequence of Corvisart's development of percussion and Laennec's invention of the stethoscope. This was the second stage of the revolution in medical theory that had begun with Bichat's brilliant studies in pathological anatomy. Symptoms, we recall Bichat saying, are incoherent phenomena, but when one opens a few corpses everything is made clear. The significance of the diagnostic revolution at La Charité was that the patient no longer had to die for the interior world of the body to brought into focus. "Auscultation and percussion," wrote a German physician, Adolf Mühry, in 1836, "make possible a kind of *living* pathological anatomy or anatomical pathology."[21] In the same spirit, as we have seen, Holmes would later describe auscultation as "that wonderful art of discovering disease, which, as it were, puts a window in the breast, through which the vital organs can be *seen*, to all intents and purposes."[22]

Holmes's first serious piece of medical writing when he returned to Boston would be his Boylston Prize essay on the set topic of direct exploration, or, in his words, "application of the sense of hearing to the direct exploration of the internal organs."[23] It was the ideal subject for a young physician newly returned from Paris. As Holmes points out, the method of percussion, although announced by Auenbrugger in 1761, entered the mainstream of medical diagnosis only with Corvisart's translation in 1808. Laennec's 1815 treatise on mediate auscultation, by the same token, was only translated by the English physician John Forbes in 1821, so that English-speaking readers have only had access to it for some fifteen years. What are the results of the new methods? They permit the physician, says Holmes, to identify early tuberculosis, and "to determine the stage and the degree of pneumonia, even when its rational signs are wanting." They reveal "the existence of pleurisies, which, clear as the day when properly sought after, have yet been long wasting the patient and perplexing the physician." In a single stroke, in short, they have "rendered the derangements of the very organs which nature seems to have barred and bolted from our reach most carefully, the best understood of all those which affect the organs of the visceral cavities."[24]

Submissions for the Boylston Prize were anonymous, the writer being identified by a Latin tag attached to the essay. The tag chosen by Holmes was *inter taedia et labores*—"amidst painful and weary labors"—the phrase Leopold Auenbrugger had used to describe the experiments leading to his Latin treatise *Inventum novum* in 1761. Auenbrugger's discovery of percussion is a twice-told tale in medical history. As the son of an innkeeper, he had often seen his father tap wine casks to determine whether they were full, empty, or partly filled. Later, as a physician at the Spanish hospital in Vienna, he realized that he could use the same method to accurately assess certain conditions within the cavity of the human chest. Like an empty wine cask, a healthy chest with properly aerated lung tissue gives back a resonant sound. Dullness, on the other hand, was a reliable sign of congestion, as in pleurisy or inflammation of the pleural sac, the serous membrane that folds back on itself to provide a frictionless envelope between the lungs and the chest wall. Less often, it might mean an abscess within the chest, with the accumulated pus explaining the dead sound (*son mat*) that expert percussionists learned to recognize through practice. As we have seen in Holmes's notes from Louis's *clinique*, it could also reveal certain pathological states of the coronary tissue.

By the time of the Paris hospital reorganization of 1794, Auenbrugger's *Inventum Novem* had become a rare curiosity of older medical literature. The origins of the school of La Charité may be traced to its rediscovery by Jean Nicolas Corvisart, who immediately recognized its extraordinary significance in the climate created by the anatomico-pathological researches of Bichat. Paradoxically, since Corvisart was a leader in the movement to abolish Latin as the language of Paris medical instruction—in part a counsel of pure practicality, since many of the students who came into the École de Médecine after the Revolution had very little Latin—his own sound classical education during the *ancien régime* permitted him to translate Auenbrugger's *Inventum Novum* into French. The translation was published in 1808. Meanwhile, Corvisart was experimenting with and perfecting Auenbrugger's method in light of the new knowledge of pathological anatomy inaugurated by Bichat's *Anatomie générale* and *Anatomie descriptive*, as well as instructing his own students in the new diagnostic technique. By 1825, as Ackerknecht remarks, the new method had spread from its center in Paris throughout the international medical community.

Nonetheless, the school of La Charité came fully into its own only with Gaspard Laurent Bayle's researches into the disease then known as *phthisis*, the terrifying "wasting disease" that the nineteenth century called consumption and that we know today as tuberculosis. Bayle was Corvisart's successor at La Charité—Corvisart had given up his academic posts to become personal physician to Napoleon—and was, like Bichat, a tireless practitioner of the new pathological anatomy. As an *interne* at La Charité, he had learned the method of percussion with which Corvisart was experimenting, and grew expert at correlating external symptoms with the lesions found at autopsy in patients who had died of phthisis. His great work, *Recherches sur la phthisie pulmonaire*, was published in 1810. Based on the results of over 900 autopsies, it gave the most detailed pathological descriptions of pulmonary tuberculosis available to that point, dividing the disease into six distinct species according to the type of lesion revealed by autopsy. Bayle died, of tuberculosis, in 1816. One of his closest friends, like him a royalist and devout Catholic, was René-Théophile-Hyacinthe Laennec.

Bayle's *Recherches sur la phthisie pulmonaire* were devoted to the disease that would elevate La Charité and its physicians to worldwide fame, the wasting or consumptive illness that, though commonly recognized in the ancient world, seemed to have gained ground during the rapid population growth of the eighteenth century. "The disease generally begins with a dry cough," wrote William Buchan in his widely-read *Domestic Medicine*, "which often continues for some months. . . . Afterwards the patient begins to spit a greenish, white, or bloody matter. . . . At last the swelling of the feet and legs, the total loss of strength, the sinking of the eyes, the difficulty of swallowing, and the coldness of the extremities, shew the immediate approach of death, which however the patient seldom believes to be so near. Such is the usual progress of this fatal disease, which . . . commonly sets all medicine at defiance."[25] Bayle's own description was at once more terse and more vivid: "In the beginning it is but a slight indisposition; at the end it floors the most vigorous individual. It devours, consumes, and reduces to a skeleton him whose belly, freshness, and health seemed unchangeable."[26] The word *phthisis*, a Greek term with the general meaning of wasting away, traces etymologically to a Greek verb that describes fuel being consumed by a fire.

The research that would allow R. T. H. Laennec to revolutionize the concept of disease in Paris medical theory began, however, with an attempt to diagnose a coronary rather than a pulmonary disorder. The story of his discovery of the stethoscope is legendary. Wanting to listen to the heart sounds of a young woman (*jeune personne*) whose buxomness hindered direct listening—and, he implies, challenged the innate modesty of the young Catholic physician ("*l'âge et le sexe de la malade m'interdisant l'espèce d'examen dont je viens de parler*")—Laennec suddenly recalled having once heard the sound of a scratching made by a needle transmitted through the entire length of a wooden beam. Rolling a notebook into a cylinder, Laennec placed it over her heart and listened. To his amazement, as he reports in a famous passage of *Auscultation médiate*, he was able to hear the sounds of the heart much more clearly than when placing his ear directly on the chest. Within a short time, the rolled-up notebook gave way to a wooden cylinder devised by Laennec himself, who was a skilled woodworker. The stethoscope, which would eventually become a symbol of the medical profession as such, was born.

The name given by Laennec to his new method of diagnosis comes from the Latin verb *auscultare*, which in one sense simply means to listen attentively, but which in classical Latin also carries strong implications of spying into secrets, as when one listens outside a door to a conversation going on in another room ("*quid habeat sermonis, auscultabo*," says a character in Plautus's *Poenulus*), and which was also used to describe domestic servants standing by to await orders. Laennec, whose Latin was excellent—he very often used Latin in his clinical teaching at La Charité, not, as was sometimes said, out of royalist nostalgia for an earlier epoch of medical teaching, but because he drew a great number of foreign students whose Latin was better than their French[27]—would have been entirely aware of these connotations. They are precisely what Holmes has in mind in speaking of auscultation, as we have heard him do, as a means of penetrating with the mind's eye "the very organs which nature seems to have barred and bolted from our reach most carefully." This was especially true, as events would show, in the case of phthisis.

The discovery for which the school of La Charité would become renowned was again Laennec's, and again the result of fortuitous accident. He was employing his new method of stethoscopic exploration on a patient whose general symptoms were those of phthisis, but whose condition had not yet been determined to be pulmonary. The episode shows exactly why what happened next would be revolutionary in its diagnostic implications. For while phthisis, a disease named after its most obvious symptoms, was very commonly associated with tubercles in the lungs, the wasting-away phenomenon might be caused by a number of other illnesses, including various forms of cancer and, more occasionally, other conditions as well. In this instance Laennec, who had a strong suspicion that the disease involved tuberculous matter in the lungs, was applying the stethoscope to various areas above the pulmonary region. When he asked the patient a question and she answered, he heard, to his amazement, that the sound seemed to be coming from the stethoscope itself: "her voice seemed to issue directly from the chest and to pass entirely up through the hole in the middle of the cylinder."[28]

Like Bichat and Corvisart and Bayle before him, Laennec was a close student of pathological anatomy, having performed innumerable autopsies on patients who had died in the final stage of pulmonary phthisis. From his own autopsies, as well as from the precise and painstaking descriptions of his friend Bayle, he was entirely familiar with what was called tubercular excavation, the empty cavity in the wall of the lung left by tubercles that had invaded the pulmonary tissue, spread to bring about the *ramolissement* or softening of a larger area of the lung, then liquefied to be evacuated through the bronchial tubes by the patient's cough, very often with the hemoptysis or bloody expectoration that was one of the most dreaded signs of tuberculosis in its final deadly stage. Now, Laennec realized, the sound of the patient's voice "inside" his stethoscope could only be due to a tubercular excavation. He named his discovery *pectoriloquy*, or "the speaking of the chest." It would become the most famous of the stethoscopic signs, a vivid example of what physicians like Mühry had in mind in speaking of auscultation as having given medicine the means of a *living* pathological anatomy, to all intents and purposes an autopsy performed while the patient was still alive.

Laennec would himself succumb to tuberculosis in 1826, in his forty-sixth year. Elisha Bartlett, later one of the most prominent exponents of Parisian medical theory in the United States, was studying in Paris at the time. "The celebrated Laennec died at his country residence on the 13th of the present month," Bartlett wrote in a letter to his sisters. "The publication in 1819 of a new method of ascertaining diseases of the chest forms an era in the history of medicine." The disease to which Laennec had fallen victim, Bartlett added, was one "the investigation of which by himself has enriched the field of science."[29] Laennec had made possible the diagnosis of many illnesses and conditions—e.g., bronchiectasis, pneumonia, emphysema, empyema—some of which he identified for the first time as separate maladies. Yet his greatest gift to the generation of Holmes and his young Boston friends was less his diagnostic method than the conception of disease to which it so insistently pointed, the notion of separate diseases as autonomous entities. Laennec's greatest gift to the Holmes who would pass through medical training to emerge as a major nineteenth-century American author, on the other hand, would be the notion of a *vis medicatrix naturae*, a healing power of nature working continuously against disease as an invasion of the body, and, in anyone who is yet alive, has so far emerged victorious.

The route by which Laennec arrived at the notion of disease as a separate entity provides part of the drama of *De l'auscultation médiate*, which is as much a story of personal discovery as a handbook of diagnosis or pathological anatomy. Laennec's friend Bayle, we recall, had after 900 autopsies managed to divide phthisis into six distinct types. He had also pronounced phthisis to be, as a disease, invariably fatal: if the patient did not proceed on a steady course to death, the illness had not been phthisis after all. In the wake of his own discovery of stethoscopic diagnosis, Laennec had found unmistakable evidence that both these points were wrong. Bayle's separate types of pulmonary phthisis—Laennec rejected several of these on the grounds that they were not tubercular in origin —were, in reality, successive stages of the same disease. The difference among them, as Laennec would famously put it, is only the difference between the same fruit at various stages of ripeness. Even today, there is a real immediacy to his descriptions of the onset and progress of tubercular lesions. The tubercles, he wrote in 1819,

> develop in the form of small semi-transparent seeds, sometimes grey, sometimes translucent and nearly colorless. Their size varies from that of a millet seed to that of a seed of hemp. In this state, one may call them *tubercles miliares* [Lat: *milius*: millet]. These seeds grow in size, becoming yellowish and opaque, first at the center, then throughout their entire mass. The ones closest to each other join together as they develop, proceeding to form a more or less extensive mass, of a pale yellow color, opaque and of the density of a firm cheese. At this stage they may be called crude tubercles (*tubercles crus*). . . . In whatever way the *tubercles crus* might have formed, they finish, at the end of a longer or shorter time, of which the duration seems to be extremely variable, by softening and liquefying. The softening begins near the center of each mass, which from day to day becomes softer and more moist, until the softening has reached the circumference of the congested tissue and may be considered complete.[30]

It is a dramatic moment. For nearly two thousand years, from well before the time of Hippocrates to the end of the eighteenth century,[31] the only story to be told about this disease was that of a patient slowly wasting away. Now there is another story, that of what Jacalyn Duffin has called "a unit lesion with a life history,"[32] oblivious to the human body it is devouring, following out to its end the grim process traced in Laennec's pathological description: infiltration, *ramolissement*, tubercular excavation, slow extinction of the capacity to process oxygen, and finally the lingering death of the patient. The matter in the tubercular excavation is a primary sign that the process is approaching its end: "sometimes it resembles a thick pus, but odorless and more yellow than the *tubercles crus.* Sometimes it is separated into two parts, one extremely liquid, more or less transparent and colorless (at least if it is not discolored by blood), the other opaque and having the consistency of soft, crumbly cheese." At this stage, the tubercular cavity eats its way through to the nearest bronchial tube, to which it remains "connected by a fistula, even after the tuberculous matter has been completely excavated."[33] The tubercular cough is now, in most cases, a sign of approaching death.

Yet Laennec's other most important discovery was that this is not always so. Bayle, in pronouncing tubercular phthisis to be invariably fatal, had been drawing his evidence exclusively from autopsies performed on subjects who had come into the hospital with symptoms of terminal consumption. It had not occurred to him, as it well might not, to look for tubercular lesions in those who had died from other ailments. Laennec, on the other hand, alerted by stethoscopic exploration to the existence of excavations in patients who had come into the hospital with other complaints, discovers to his amazement that some of them have progressed to the second stage of tubercular infection and then, spontaneously as it might be, have gotten better. "From time to time one finds," he reports, "in the bodies of those who have suffered from a chronic catarrh, and who have died from one or another malady, cavities with a jagged rim that are lined by a semi-cartilaginous membrane, exactly like that which lines old ulcers in the lung, which these cavities resemble in every respect, except that they contain not the least trace of tuberculous matter."[34] In these empty cavities, says Laennec, one finds a scarlike tissue where the *ramolissement* had earlier taken place. The lung has healed, and, though somewhat compromised, has given no further trouble.

Laennec's reasoning from the evidence of these empty and cicatrized cavities is a model of diagnostic inference. In patients who have died after a long period of consumption, autopsy reveals old excavations, very much like those in these recovered patients, alongside more recent ones. When the physician carefully interrogates patients who come into the hospital with a chronic catarrh, no matter what complaint has actually brought them in, one normally finds that they can trace their cough to a serious illness earlier in life, one that "presented all the symptoms of pulmonary phthisis, often to such a degree that, at the time of the illness, one would have diagnosed them as hopeless cases of chest disease."[35] More dramatically, one can discover in the bodies of recently-deceased tuberculous patients a membrane that has begun to close over the surface of more advanced cavities—the very membrane that, when the cavity has been evacuated, is transformed into what Laennec calls a sort of internal scar tissue (*cicatrice interne*) that seals off the injured portion of the lung. "The formation of this semi-cartilaginous membrane on the surface of tuberculous ulcers," says Laennec, "ought, it seems to me, to be taken as an effort made by the healing power of nature (*la nature médicatrice*).[36]

As we shall see, the notion of a "Parisian" school in nineteenth-century American medicine has constant reference to the new conception of disease as an autonomous entity. It was resisted by physicians trained in the older humoral pathology. Auscultation, as the symbol of the new theory, would at first be met with outright derision. Even devotees of the new diagnostic method could understand why. There is, admitted John Forbes, Laennec's first English translator, something ludicrous in the picture of a grave physician listening attentively to a long tube applied to the patient's chest, "as if the disease were a living being that could communicate its condition to the sense without."[37] Yet the clinical evidence, constantly accumulating as more and more physicians grew expert in the method, would demonstrate that the stethoscope put the doctor in possession of a truth unknown to the patient. "Even excavations in the lungs," Holmes would serenely insist in his Boylston Prize essay, "may precede the existence of either cough or expectoration; and they are found in the bodies of patients who have died of various diseases, and in whom no thoracic symptoms have excited attention."[38]

In the same essay, the consequences for medical authority are made dramatically clear in a passage Holmes cites from Charles J. B. Williams's *Rational Exposition of the Physical Signs of the Diseases of the Lungs and Pleura* (1828), the first systematic treatise on the new internal pathology to appear in English. Dr. Williams is describing pectoriloquy, that "speaking of the chest" that Laennec had discovered by accident: "'More than once has it occurred to me that the very words, which in that delusive confidence with which this malady enshrouds its victims, ridiculed my examination of the chest, roundly saying, that nothing ailed them there, have belied their meaning, and coming from the breast, have told a far different tale!' "[39] The grim irony emerges even through the Victorian embellishments of Williams's diction. The patient, sure that he is in robust overall health, loudly protests that stethoscopic exploration is a waste of time. Simultaneously the doctor, hearing these same words ascend to him directly through the stethoscope, understands that he is listening to a tubercular excavation declaring, like some grinning skull in a medieval woodcut, that this particular patient's days on earth are numbered.

Such episodes were taken, by Holmes and other Paris-trained American physicians, as conclusive evidence that genuine medical authority could proceed only from the systematic study and adequate clinical instruction that put the doctor in possession of a diagnostic truth unavailable to the patient. This is the view that would sustain Holmes, in subsequent years, in his strenuous combat against homeopathy and the varieties of medical quackery that flourished under the conditions of Jacksonian democracy.[40] It is what he has in mind in telling his parents in an early letter from Paris that, in a wholly unparadoxical sense, he already has far more medical experience than many a gray-haired practitioner in their own neighborhood. For the young Parisian medical student "has been instructed daily . . . by men who know no master and teach no doctrine but Nature and her laws, pointed out at the bedside for those to own who see them . . . ; he has examined the dead body more often and more thoroughly in the course of a year than the vast majority of our practitioners have in any ten years of their lives. True experience is the product of opportunity multiplied by years."[41]

In recent years, some medical historians, writing from the perspective of such "people's doctors" as the botanical practitioner Samuel Thomson, have tried to demystify claims like those Holmes is making here as being due to nothing more than anxieties of "professionalization." A later essay such as Holmes's *Homeopathy and Its Kindred Delusions* would not, on their view, testify to any genuine concern for medical truth or patient welfare, being only the attempt of a certain professional cohort to assert its claims against others competing in the marketplace. Yet to such younger physicians as Holmes and William Gerhard and James Jackson, Jr. the notion of medical truth was very real, something to be asserted in the same spirit as a Galileo or Newton had asserted their theories of the physical universe, truth that matters not because it serves the professional ambitions of this or that investigator, but because it is true. There is no other way to make sense, it seems to me, of the emphasis placed by younger American physicians of the "Paris school" on systematic and first-hand anatomico-pathological experience, which in their own case necessarily meant having been present in person in Paris. The essence of their claims is caught in a dictum of Gaspard-Laurent Bayle's that Chomel liked to quote to his students: "There is in the art of diagnosis, as in prognosis, something that cannot be transmitted by words nor by writings."[42]

Exploration by percussion and auscultation provides a perfect illustration of their point. John Forbes, as we have seen, undertook a translation of Laennec's *De l'auscultation médiate* that was meant to add to the vocabulary of English-speaking physicians equivalents of the various technical terms—*pectoriloquie, bronchophonie, Égophonie (résonnance chevrotante), râle trachéale, râle muqueux, râle crépitant humide, râle sous-crépitant, tintement métallique,* etc.—given to the sounds heard by students of Laennec or Chomel or Louis. Like the Paris doctors, Forbes tried to make such terms intelligible by comparing them to sounds heard in the everyday world. Hippocrates, in an example that the proponents of percussion and auscultation never tired of claiming as a precedent, had compared the sound of liquid in a patient's chest as being like the sound of boiling vinegar. In the same spirit, Chomel would compare *tintement métallique* as being "like a drop of water falling into a metallic vase," and the *râle crepitant*, a sign of pneumonia, as being like "the tearing of a taffeta."[43]

If the new diagnostic techniques could be learned from a book, in short, Forbes's *Treatise on Diseases of the Chest* ought to have put practitioners in London or New York or Kentucky on a par with those accompanying Laennec or Chomel on rounds at La Charité. But in fact the analogies given by the Paris teachers were a prime example of the failure of language, as such, to connect with sensory perception: the classical philosophical problem of trying to describe the taste of a pineapple to someone who has never tasted one. Chomel's "drop of water falling into a metallic vase" made sense only to students who were able to hear what he himself had just heard, and even then was not an easy sound to distinguish when one was still learning. The difficulty explains a certain note of frustration in Mason Warren's letters—"in *Catarrhe Pulmonaire*," he patiently explains to his father, " a *subcrepitant rale* is heard at the lower part of the chest"[44]—and the note of pure exhilaration in James Jackson, Jr.'s voice as he tells his own father that he has learned to hear bronchial respiration:

> I heard it last summer in several cases in Andral's ward, during the second stage of pneumonia; and from him I learned to distinguish it from vesicular respiration. I remember well one case, in which he said you will hear upon the right side the bronchial respiration at the same time with the vesicular, and on the other the bronchial alone. I listened, and could make this distinction; was confident of it. The difference consisted in a slow expansion of the vesicles by the air in the one, and an absence of this in the other.[45]

The source of Jackson's exhilaration is the Paris discovery of what Jacalyn Duffin has called anatomico-pathological correlation. No amount of listening through the stethoscope could reveal the slow expansion of vesicles that Jackson is describing. It is necessary to have examined those vesicles in a hundred autopsies, then to be able to visualize them as they exist in the living body. This is what Chomel meant, for instance, in trying to get across to students the distinction between a mere *symptom* and a diagnostic *sign*, which was an event in the mind of the trained observer. The sign, he said, is "a phenomenon perceptible to the senses, which leads to knowledge of more hidden facts. It is a conclusion that the mind [*l'esprit*] draws from the symptom, while the symptom is simply a perception. The one pertains more to the judgment, the other to the senses.

The symptom is appreciable to all the world. The physician alone can discover the signs within the symptoms."[46] Holmes had the same point in mind when, addressing an audience of medical students many years later, he would tell them that the *tactus eruditus*, the physical touch of the learned physician, "extends to the mind as well as to the finger-ends."[47]

On the other hand, the same diagnostic expertise could create a sense of utter helplessness in the trained physician. Consider, for instance, the famous phenomenon of the *spes phthisica*, which was the sense of unreal or delusive optimism experienced by tuberculosis patients on the very threshold of death. "What is most wonderful," reported an ancient medical writer, "is that in a case when blood comes from the lung, in which the disease is most serious, patients do not give up hope."[48] The *spes phthisica* is what Buchan is talking about when he remarks in *Domestic Medicine* that tubercular patients even in their extremity seldom believe death to be near, and what we have heard Dr. Williams describe as the "delusive confidence with which this malady enshrouds its victims." More dramatically than anything else, the encounter with *spes phthisica* would throw into sharp relief for Holmes the helplessness of the physician who knows that a patient is very near to death, but who is unable to do anything to alter the course of the disease. In later years, as a professor at Harvard, he would always make it a point to warn medical students just entering into practice that they must never permit the patient to glimpse their own sense of futility:

> No matter how hard he stares at your countenance, he should never be able to read his fate in it. It should be cheerful as long as there is hope, and serene in its gravity when nothing is left but resignation. The face of a physician, like that of a diplomatist, should be impenetrable. Nature is a benevolent old hypocrite; she cheats the sick and the dying with illusions better than any anodynes. If there are cogent reasons why a patient should be undeceived, do it deliberately and advisedly, but do not betray your apprehensions through your tell-tale features.[49]

"It is a terrible thing," he tells them a bit later, "to take away hope, even earthly hope, from a fellow-creature."[50]

A partial answer to this dilemma, as we shall see, would be found by Paris-trained physicians in the *méthode expectante*, the practice of doing everything possible to aid nature in the process of recovery from disease, and to do nothing to hinder what we have heard Laennec, taking over into French the Latin phrase *vis medicatrix naturae*, call *la nature médi-catrice* —no small accomplishment in the day when physicians, backed by a thousand years of Galenic or humoral medicine, were trained to attack disease vigorously with bleeding, emetics, purgatives, blisters, and a myriad other ostensible remedies meant, as the American physician Benjamin Rush would put it, to drive Nature, clearly in a disordered state at present, out the door. Still, medicine since the time of Hippocrates had been based on the idea of the physician as a healer. A new medical theory able to offer precise diagnosis but no remedy for disease was extremely vulnerable on the point of its self-confessed powerlessness in the area of therapy. This would be the primary basis of the attack on Laennec and the school of La Charité by its fiercest opponent, the dynamic and violently controversial chief physician of the Val de Grâce, François Joseph Victor Broussais, advocate of the opposing school of what he would call "physiological medicine."

To historians of medicine, Broussais's attack on Laennec is noteworthy primarily as a turning point in the emergence of Paris anatomico-pathological theory. As regards the relation between Holmes's Paris medical education and his career as an American writer, however, the episode is far more important for having given visibility to what John Harley Warner has described as "therapeutic stagnation"—what I have called the therapeutic hiatus in nineteenth-century medicine—whose beginning was marked by Bichat's pioneering researches in pathological anatomy.[51] Broussais's attack on Laennec made painfully clear to everyone associated with the school of La Charité that its achievement involved an undeniable paradox. At a time when diagnosis had attained great exactness, and when the nature of disease was better understood than at any previous time in human history, no Paris physician was a bit better than his Greek or Roman or Renaissance counterpart at doing anything about the illness he had so confidently identified. The consequences for Holmes's later career as a medical writer, and then as author of the Breakfast Table books, would be, as we shall see, significant.

Broussais's popularity as a teacher was due partly to the achievements of his early career. As someone who had dared to attack Pinel's immensely influential *Nosographie* on the grounds of its "ontologism"— i.e., its attempt to elevate mere constellations of symptoms into "diseases in themselves"—he had cleared the way for the subsequent correlation of external symptoms with internal lesions for which Paris medicine would become famous. As the self-appointed inheritor of Bichat's localism and solidism, which he saw himself as having radicalized by tracing the origin of most diseases to inflammation of the gastro-intestinal tract, he was a plausible candidate for the throne of anatomico-pathological medicine left vacant by Bichat's untimely death. And, as Braunstein's recent *Broussais et le matérialisme* persuasively demonstrates, he was able to promote his "physiological medicine" as being in essential harmony with the doctrines that had contributed so powerfully to the French Revolution. This is, once again, Holbach and the La Mettrie of *L'homme machine* as lying in the immediate philosophical background of the Paris medical revolution.

Another source of Broussais's immense authority during the period that he dominated Paris medicine was the therapeutic regimen he introduced as the corollary of his theories of gastro-intestinal inflammation. For while Laennec, having carefully described tubercular excavations or hepatized lung tissue, was then unable to alleviate, let alone cure, either pulmonary phthisis or pneumonia, Broussais provided not only a therapy but an explanation of why it worked. The explanation was his doctrine of irritation, an updated version of the "excitability" that the eighteenth-century Scottish physician John Brown, himself updating an older humoralism, had made the central physiological principle involved in all disease. Living tissues respond to external stimuli—or, in Broussais's physiological medicine, such psychological causes as stress, anger, or depression—in a way that, in ordinary circumstances, permits normal function of the organism, but that in extraordinary circumstances brings about the imbalance that we call illness or disease. For Brown, still operating largely in the terms of humoral imbalance, the consequence was either an "sthenic" or "asthenic" state, a disorder resulting either from too great or too little excitation. For Broussais, it was inflammation, and in most cases inflammation of the gastrointestinal system.

The solution to inflammation was bleeding, a primary remedy used in the older humoral medicine, but now revised by Broussais to suit the demands of his own radical localism. The traditional means of bleeding the patient had been venesection, or cutting open a vein to let the blood spill into a basin, cupping, a technique for drawing blood by inverting and heating a specially designed glass vessel over an incision, or by use of leeches, the blood-sucking aquatic worms so commonly used in the medieval period that *leech* became an Old English synonym for "physician." Broussais's innovation was to popularize bloodletting by leeches, conceived as a local rather than general remedy, as a measure to be used against the local inflammations posited by his theory. In older histories of Paris medicine, the popularity of Broussais's physiological doctrines was sometimes demonstrated by charts or tables displaying the balance of the French leech trade, which went from the exportation of a million leeches in 1820 to the net importation of forty million in 1833, the year Holmes arrived in Paris. Broussais's *médecine physiologique* could thus at once be perceived as radically new, a logical development of Bichat's anatomico-pathological discoveries, and comfortingly traditional.

Another explanation of Broussais's enormous influence, however, was his personal dynamism, and not least his ability to hold spellbound the thousands of students who flocked to the military hospital at the Val de Grâce to hear the apostle of the new physiological medicine announce his latest findings and triumphantly declare their superiority to the claims of every competing medical theory, ancient and modern. This is the voice one may still hear, for instance, in Broussais's *Examen des Doctrines Médicales*, as when he explains why, not having been privy to the principles of his own physiological system, even so great a pathologist as Morgagni had been sadly deficient in essential insight:

> To discover the faults in the work of this author, it is absolutely necessary to have been enlightened by physiology. For it is this [*la physiologie*] that makes us aware of those things we have sought for in vain in the writings of ancient and modern authors. It teaches us that an inflammation of the stomach, which only shows itself through mild discomfort in the epigastrium, or on one or the other side of the hypochondrium, is able to cause, through a system of sympathetic communication, those disturbances in which one might be tempted to attribute death to an illness [*affection*] of the brain or spinal extension. It is by it that we know that all gastrointestinal irritations are repeated by the secretory portions of the liver, from which one easily draws the conclusion that they are able to bring about a derangement of tissues [*désorganisation*]; so that a jaundiced liver, streaked or marbled, is always connected to an inflammation of the duodenum [*une duodénite*] or of the middle portion of the small intestine.[52]

The story of Broussais's attack on Laennec is one of the least attractive chapters in the history of Paris medicine, but essential nonetheless for understanding the context in which American students like Holmes and James Jackson, Jr. and William Gerhard would absorb the teachings of P. C. A. Louis in the wards of La Pitié. As Jacalyn Duffin has pointed out in a perceptive essay, Broussais and Laennec at a deep level shared a certain skepticism about the new localism and solidism of the Bichatian anatomico-pathological school. For Broussais, the whole point of his physiological medicine—that is, a medicine that looked beyond lesions to the derangement of organic *function* that caused them, as when stress or other causes induced gastrointestinal inflammation—was to provide a theoretical context for findings like those of Bichat. For Laennec, on the other hand, one clear implication of the new conception of disease as an autonomous entity was, precisely, that it included illnesses that could not be traced to anatomical lesions. To perform an autopsy on someone who had suffered from malaria, for instance—the dread "intermittent fever" that had ruined the health of so many in both the ancient and modern worlds—was to find, in the way of local lesions, nothing at all.

As a contest of personalities, the combat between Broussais and Laennec was an unequal match. For Broussais, robust, ebullient, overflowing with aggressive energy, was a magnetic personality in both the clinic and the lecture room. Laennec, stooped, emaciated, and already weakened by the tuberculosis that would eventually kill him, was a hesitant public speaker and a tentative personality even in the more intimate setting of the clinic. Yet Laennec would emerge victorious from the contest, not least because Broussais made the major miscalculation of carrying the vituperative mode of his classroom lectures over into the *Examen*. Thus, for instance, he will not only denounce Laennec for denying that pneumonia alters the size or volume of the lungs—which Broussais maintains that it does—but proceeds to an ad hominem attack. M. Laennec, he remarks with unmistakable sarcasm, has written that "*a doctor who has the habit of supporting his opinions with a great deal of warmth, told him that he had several times found hepatized lungs on which an imprint of the ribs had been made*, but he believes that the *memory* or the *eyes* of this doctor *have deceived him*, because he (M. L[aennec]) *has never seen any such thing.*"[53]

Broussais, as he well knows, is the physician Laennec was talking about. He rises instantly to the bait. Having made a perfectly good logical point in passing—"To deny a fact because one has never seen it personally, is hardly the part of a wise man"—he then proceeds to a marshaling of anecdotal evidence. Not only has Broussais himself seen the imprint of the ribs on the tissue of a lung, but his colleague M. Peysson, physician of the military hospital at Cambray, has written him about a similar case: "'at the autopsy of a man who had died of a longtime pleurisy with discharge, I encountered the imprint of the ribs on the lungs themselves. There were other witnesses present whose attention I directed to this singular phenomenon, while saying to them that Dr. Laennec had been wrong to deny this fact against a colleague whom he does not name'." Might Dr. Peysson just perhaps have recognized him as the person Laennec was talking about, asks Broussais with heavy sarcasm, "from the *warmth of my opinions?*" If so, there is nothing wrong with supporting one's opinions warmly, so long as they are backed up by facts: "so many men today take a frigid attitude towards truth, that I am hardly about to reject being praised for having pled her cause with some warmth."[54]

In both the *Examen* and his lectures at the Val de Grâce and the École de Médecine, Broussais epitomizes an aspect of the Paris medical revolution to which historians have only recently begun to pay serious attention: the essential theatricality of the setting in which the Paris doctors presented their theories, defended their procedures, and combated rival claims.[55] This was sufficiently remarked at the time, very often with reference to Broussais. "With more knowledge of books and ideas," wrote the medical journalist Louis Peisse in 1827, "with convictions that were acquired more industriously and conscientiously, with distinction and taste, he would probably have moved the medical masses less. Great popularity is only acquired at the price of a certain vulgarity. Perhaps without these brutalities, the partial truth and common sense which formed the strength of his polemic would not have penetrated into the minds of the majority. He would not have created a revolution."[56] Howard Payson Arnold, author of an invaluable and neglected memoir of Mason Warren, captures a sense of the same spirit as it animated the great Paris surgeons:

> One was reminded of a band of gladiators fiercely contending, Paris serving as their arena, and the whole globe as their amphitheatre. . . . Their inordinate eagerness to dazzle and captivate by nimble *tours de main* and theatrical *éclat*, and thus to impress mankind with a sense of their superiority, was indescribable. From this resulted a frightful loss of life, as the patient was often sacrificed to the splendor of the operation. . . . They cut up their victims as they cut up each other, cruelly, recklessly; and death brought a welcome repose to those whom they sacrificed.[57]

This theatricality is another element of Holmes's Paris medical training that would have enormous influence on his subsequent career as a popular Lyceum lecturer, reciter of his own verse on public occasions, and, most significantly, the self-dramatized personality whose voice the world would first hear in *The Autocrat of the Breakfast Table*. Yet the deeper impact of such teachers as Chomel, Andral, and Louis would be to establish in his mind two separate categories of truth: a truth of opinion or public sentiment, essential to civic existence and legitimately upheld in literary or rhetorical terms, and a truth of external or physical nature in relation to which rhetoric or theatricality were utterly irrelevant. Holmes's lifelong sense of scientific truth as something immune to rhetorical manipulation traces back, ultimately, to the lessons he learned as a student in the school of La Charité. For what would account for Laennec's ultimate victory over Broussais was not a superiority in vituperation, but the inexorable spread of the stethoscopic method itself. Every young doctor who purchased a stethoscope and learned to hear the distinctive sounds of the *râle sous-crépitant* or the *tintement métallique* was, in effect, entering the battle on the side of Laennec and the conception of disease as an autonomous entity.

By the time Holmes himself arrived in Paris, the contest was essentially over, even though, in the years after Laennec's death, Broussais would futilely try to restore the prestige of his *médecine physiologique* by turning his verbal artillery on P. C. A. Louis, by then emerging as the new luminary of the school of La Charité. Holmes's own description of Broussais lecturing during this period has been widely quoted in histories of Paris medicine. It is nonetheless worth quoting once more. The fiery old theorist, as Holmes calls him, continued to teach at the

École de Médecine, unwilling to admit that his theory was now widely regarded as having been exploded. "The hour of his lecture," recalls Holmes, "was succeeded by that of a younger and far more popular professor. As his lecture drew towards its close, the benches, thinly sprinkled with students, began to fill up; the doors creaked open and banged back oftener and oftener, until at last the sound grew almost continuous, and the voice of the lecturer became a leonine growl as he strove in vain to be heard over the noise of doors and footsteps."[58]

The younger lecturer who attracted such a crowd of students was Gabriel Andral, whose course in Internal Pathology Holmes attended during the winter of 1833 and the spring of 1834. To these students, the special appeal of Andral's teaching was that, although he had clearly mastered the lessons of the Paris anatomico-pathological revolution, including the important discoveries of Corvisart and Laennec at La Charité, his restless intelligence was already at work attempting to give precise formulation to medical problems that could not be resolved by the correlation of symptoms with anatomical lesions. He was, moreover, a brilliant teacher. "The glory of the week," James Jackson, Jr. wrote to his father in November, 1832, "has been Andral's introductory lecture. . . . It was the most eloquent I ever heard, one speech of Mr Webster's and a sermon or two of Dr Channing's excepted. I could scarcely restrain myself, it was so grand and beautiful. What powers of mind and vastness of comprehension has this man! What gave me peculiar pleasure also, he declared boldly and freely for the numerical method, saying, it was the only mode of advancing the science of pathology."[59]

Together with Chomel and Louis, whom he had gotten to know at La Charité, Andral was a principal figure in the reign of "eclecticism," the last period of Paris medicine and, in the estimate of Erwin Ackerknecht, "probably the richest and most brilliant period of them all."[60] The usefulness of the term eclecticism may be doubted. Borrowed from the philosopher Victor Cousin, who was a patient of Laennec's, a friend of Andral's, and a defender of the principles of the Restoration, it was adopted as a slogan during the tumultuous course of French politics after the fall of Napoleon. Laennec had adopted the term to describe his own medical approach, but this was no doubt, as Jacalyn Duffin suggests, with the mischievous intention of provoking the old revolutionary Broussais.[61] So far as it meant anything specific when applied to medical theory, it would presumably imply a determination to take the best of the old along with the best of the new—an uncontroversial stance, but one that scarcely explains the exalted note of intellectual urgency so obvious in James Jackson, Jr.'s account of Andral's lecture.

A better name for the position shared by this last generation of La Charité physicians would be skeptical empiricism—a commitment not simply to retaining the principles of empirical investigation initiated by Bichat, but then to ruthlessly and systematically jettisoning anything that did not meet the same exacting standards. Their position bears a certain resemblance to that made famous by Karl Popper in *The Logic of Scientific Discovery*, the notion that objective inquiry proceeds not by moving towards some defined solution—for the solution to the problem is always, by definition, so far unknown—but through falsification, the systematic elimination of mistaken hypotheses. In one of his later medical essays, Holmes would come very close to summing up the spirit that animated researchers like Louis and lecturers like Andral during his own Paris medical education: "Science is the topography of ignorance. From a few elevated points we triangulate vast spaces, inclosing infinite unknown details. We cast the lead, and draw up a little sand from abysses we may never reach. . . . The best part of our knowledge is that which teaches us where knowledge leaves off and ignorance begins."[62]

Holmes's Boylston Prize essay on direct exploration testifies to his allegiance to the school of La Charité not simply in giving a detailed account of percussion and auscultation as diagnostic methods instituted by Corvisart and Laennec, but because it then also demonstrates throughout so clear a conception of disease as an autonomous entity. The disease that had always previously been called phthisis, for instance, is designated by Holmes "tubercular phthisis," important evidence that, for Paris-trained physicians like himself, the transition from an older humoral medicine to the new anatomico-pathological view is nearly complete. For as historians of Paris medicine have pointed out, one of the most important signs of the epistemological revolution that had started with Bichat is a steady tendency to rename diseases always before known by their symptoms—in the case of chest diseases, for instance,"fever, difficulty breathing, cough, wheezing, spitting blood, pain, and palpitations"[63]—after the anatomical lesions discovered at autopsy. The alteration of diagnostic terminology from *phthisis*—the slow wasting away experienced by the patient—to *tuberculosis*—a name taken from the tubercle as physical sign—is the history of the Paris medical revolution writ small.

Yet the skeptical empiricism of the school of La Charité was not reserved for the older verities of Galenic humoralism, or for such modern excursions into premature speculation as Broussais's gastrointestinal theory of disease. Consider, for instance, the spirit of the dispute, amply treated by Holmes in his Boylston essay, over the stethoscopic sign of bronchophony (*bronchophonie*). This was a controversy within the school of La Charité itself, a challenge to the great Laennec by younger physicians who had eagerly adopted his method of stethoscopic exploration. They were now coming up with results that carried Laennec's work into

Oliver Wendell Holmes in Paris

new areas, with the unsettling implication that the master had only partially understood the promise of his own discovery. The controversy was extremely complicated—I refer the reader to Duffin's superb reconstruction of its details in *To See With a Better Eye*[64]—but its essence lay in the fact that pectoriloquy, that "speaking of the chest" that Laennec had correctly identified with tubercular excavations, had been discovered to be a sign as well of hepatized pulmonary tissue, that liver-like consistency of the lung that is still taken today as a primary effect of second-stage pneumonia. When the phenomenon was first pointed out to him, Laennec flatly refused to accept it as true pectoriloquy.

His refusal may have had to do with injured amour propre, an unwillingness to admit that he, the discoverer of auscultation, had missed something as crucial as the sign of terminal disease in a common illness. But as Duffin points out, there were heavy diagnostic stakes involved as well. For Laennec had put a great deal of emphasis, in reporting his results, on the Hippocratic distinction between *symptômes propres*—those that were unique to a single disease, like tubercular excavations in the case of pulmonary phthisis—and *symptômes communes*, those that, like fever, were common to many illnesses.[65] It was by not recognizing this distinction, Laennec thought, that Pinel had created such elaborate forms of nonsense as his "essential fevers." The same distinction was no doubt what he was trying to preserve in insisting on a one-to-one correlation between pectoriloquy and tubercular excavations. So it was that Laennec would try to maintain that the sound perceived in the case of hepatized lung tissue was really bronchophony, a form of "imperfect" pectoriloquy that the experienced clinician could learn to recognize by a sound transmitted only part way up the stethoscope.

The problem was that no one else could hear the difference. In his Boylston essay, Holmes treats with amused detachment the claims of the great inventor of auscultation: "To speak of the tones of the voice being heard a *short distance up the stethoscope* . . . is to present the student a distinction of such tenuity as must seem beyond the reach of his faculties. That his doctrines have led into error I am confident. The fallacy of pectoriloquy as a positive sign of the existence of caverns, is shown by its occasional presence in consequence of hepatization." Since the point is still considered controversial by some, Holmes introduces two authorities in support of his own position. One is Andral: "'by the sole fact of considerable induration of the pulmonary tissue, the voice may present a resonance more or less resembling that of perfect pectoriloquy.'" The other is Chomel: "'Pectoriloquy may exist in different degrees of tubercular disease, pulmonary induration, and effusion.'"[66] It does seem as if the inventor of auscultation, concludes Holmes, "in his anxiety to uphold the constant coincidence between pectoriloquy and pulmonary excavations, had somewhat forgotten the principles which he commonly followed with such rigor."[67]

When he wrote these words, Holmes was 26 years old. He had been awarded his M.D. from Harvard only five months before. Yet the note of self-confident certainty one catches in his voice is not egotism or arrogance, but a simple allegiance to the spirit of skeptical empiricism he had brought back from Paris. As Laennec had shown no hesitation about correcting the errors of his friend Bayle when the stethoscope opened up new possibilities in pathological anatomy, and as Chomel and Andral had not hesitated to correct Laennec himself when he attempted to save his favorite principle of *symptômes propres* by inventing a stethoscopic sign that no one else could hear, the young Holmes is perfectly willing to stake his claims in the Boylston essay on the results of his own experience with living patients and dead bodies. Nor are Holmes's citations of Andral and Chomel—the citation of Chomel is to "MS. notes," which could only be Chomel's Paris clinical lectures as attended by Holmes—a mere empty display of "Parisian" authority. Their intent is to demonstrate that, as we have heard Holmes say in a letter to his parents, the writer of this essay has been studying with teachers "who know no master and teach no doctrine but Nature and her laws."

Read in this light, Holmes's notebook from Andral's lectures in internal pathology may be taken as a virtual guide to Paris medicine in its self-denominated period of eclecticism. For Andral smoothly incorporates every element of real knowledge that has so far emerged from the researches of anatomico-pathological medicine, as when he gives in passing what amounts to a compressed summary of Laennec's *Auscultation Médiate:* "Tubercle.—Slightly yellowish-white—roundish—of variable form—. . . softens later, and transforms itself into two different matters—one white & swimming in a serous fluid—. . . It leaves a cavity, which may become larger, smaller and cicatrize; or remain the same."[68] But much more of his presentation is devoted to isolating problems to which no anatomical lesions may be shown to correspond, as when Andral points out that Broussais's doctrine of gastrointestinal inflammation must be stretched to the breaking point to account for diseases like malaria: "He has neglected the <u>general diseases</u>. In explaining secondary general diseases he has thrown the process upon <u>sympathy</u> only. The <u>blood</u> may be and is in certain cases the medium. . . .—I believe his method of accounting for intermittent fevers is erroneous."[69]

Andral's emphasis on unresolved problems is no doubt why anyone familiar with Holmes's career as medical writer discovers, in reading through these notes, so many clear anticipations of his own later preoccupations. Thus, to choose just one example, Andral, using an older vocabulary of clinical observation, will ponder the problem of what he calls puerperal diathesis: some women after childbirth come down with an infectious disease and die. Others do not. What explains the difference? Or, to consider a closely-related problem, what, exactly, is contagion? Holmes's transcription: "Different diseases may originate—first for those confined—second for those who subsequently come among them. . . . hospital gangrene.—. . . Other effects proceeding from the same cause—peritonitis in puerperal women in public establishments—attended with great prostration." Then, in an uncanny premonition of the intuition that a few years later would descend upon both Semmelweis and Holmes himself: "Different ways in which contagion may arrive—1st. contact—the skin remaining whole—or the epidermis broken—2. The mucous membranes—3. Contact of dead bodies."[70]

Some ten years after Holmes was jotting these notes in the grand lecture hall at the École de Médecine, his friend Elisha Bartlett would write him to announce that he had just composed, for an American readership, a treatise on Parisian medical theory. Their friendship dated from the days when they had been colleagues on the faculty of Dartmouth Medical School, to which Holmes had been called as a Professor of Anatomy in 1839. In later years, it was sustained not only by their appreciation of each others' wit and intelligence, but also by a sense of shared allegiance to a notion of medical authority commanding less and less assent in an age of homeopathy and hydropathy and Thomsonian botanical practitioners. "I have attempted a pretty full, and elaborate developement [sic] of what I conceive to be the true nature and philosophy of medical science,—so generally, according to my notions, either very partially and loosely apprehended, or altogether and totally mis-apprehended, and misunderstood. . . ," Bartlett wrote. "My doctrines, I am well aware, will encounter—if they are considered of importance enough to attract any considerable degree of notice—strong opposition, and I shall look to you as one of the few men disposed and qualified to stand by them."[71]

The title of Bartlett's treatise was *An Essay on the Philosophy of Medicine.* It was, declared no less an authority than Erwin Ackerknecht, "the only systematic formulation of the great Paris clinical school," so compelling as to merit Bartlett the title of the philosopher of Paris medicine.[72] The aim of his essay was, Bartlett told Holmes, "to vindicate and restore the empirical philosophy, in all its purity and absoluteness; and to exhibit the true character of all dogmatisms, rationalisms, and a priorisms—the evil genius of our science."[73] To read the *Essay* today is, for those familiar with Holmes's own Paris studies, to hear the voices of the physicians of La Charité echoing in the background. Paris medicine, wrote Bartlett, "is characterized by its strict adherence to the study and analysis of morbid phenomena and their relationships; by the accuracy, the positiveness, and the minute detail which it has carried into this study and analysis; and by its rejection as an essential or legitimate element of science of all *a priori* reasoning or speculation. . . . It is the true *protestant* school of medicine. It either rejects as apocryphal, or holds as of no binding authority, all the traditions of the fathers, unless they are sustained and sanctioned by its own experience."[74]

The glory of the Paris clinical school has been, from this perspective, its success in clearing away the rubbish of the past, putting an end to an age-old humoral pathology based on little more than the primitive speculations of Greek physics, as well as fearlessly challenging the pretensions of *a priori* systems devised by such modern writers as Cullen and Brown and Broussais. This was the side of the battle into which Holmes would enter in his later polemics against homeopathy and, more occasionally and obliquely, the ignorant "people's doctors" given to attacking regularly-educated physicians in the languages of an increasingly self-assertive Jacksonian democracy. Yet the purely negative or skeptical tendency within Paris medicine would never, by itself, have commanded the allegiance even of such remorselessly logical souls as Elisha Bartlett and Oliver Wendell Holmes. The secret of their allegiance lay, rather, in a conviction that the essence of Paris clinical training lay not simply in its power to explode old or dangerous systems, but in the promise it seemed to hold out of opening the way to as-yet-uncharted regions of medical truth.

For the young Bostonians studying with Holmes at the École de Médecine, the person who symbolized that promise was Pierre Charles Alexander Louis, a shy individual whose exceptional talents as a clinical researcher were cast into the shade by more dynamic personalities like Chomel and Andral. Yet these colleagues understood the importance of Louis's investigations. "He declared boldly and freely for the numerical method," we recall James Jackson, Jr., telling his father about Andral, "saying, it was the only mode of advancing the science of pathology." Young Jackson would become a disciple of Louis's numerical method. "Had medicine been studied for one hundred years, as Louis now studies it," said Jackson somewhat later, "our knowledge of the natural history of disease would be placed upon an infinitely more certain basis; and diagnosis, and prognosis, and consequently therapeutics vastly more advanced."[75] For young physicians like William Gerhard, the influence of Louis would inspire researches that would begin to put American medicine on a par with Europe. For Oliver Wendell Holmes, especially in the period leading up to *The Autocrat of the Breakfast Table*, it would inspire a metaphysics of rational consciousness that provided a grand alternative to the blind material universe proclaimed by nineteenth-century science.

CHAPTER THREE

The Clinic of Dr. Louis

*I*n an essay written over a century ago, Sir William Osler drew attention to the extraordinary influence exerted on an entire generation of American medical students by Pierre Charles Alexandre Louis, a modest, reticent, even shy clinical researcher at the outlying Parisian hospital of La Pitié. The group included Oliver Wendell Holmes and his Harvard friends James Jackson, Jr., Mason Warren, and Henry Bowditch. Of all the Americans who during the nineteenth century "sought light and learning in the older lands," wrote Osler, the "young men who studied in Paris, between 1830 and 1840, had no predecessors and have had no successors. Partly because the time was ripe and they were active agents in bringing the new art and science to the New World, partly owing to inherent capabilities, but not a little because the brightest minds among them fell under the influence of Louis—they more than any others gave an impetus, which it still feels, to the scientific study of medicine in the United States."[1] In light of more recent studies in the history of medicine it has begun to seem important to raise a question Osler himself never thought of addressing. Why did Louis have so great an impact on, specifically, American students?

The letters and memoirs of Americans studying in Paris at the time make it clear that his influence had nothing to do with personal charisma. Quite the reverse. Louis was, as Henry Bowditch would recall some forty years later, "ill at ease in the teacher's chair. He would talk fluently by the bedside of a patient, and give out the brilliant results of his years of patient labors in Chomel's wards, but he was awkward with his notes when lecturing. . . . The consequence of all this was that Louis always had few followers. 'He was dry,' the students said."[2] Holmes strikes a similar note in "Some of My Early Teachers," the talk given to his last anatomy class at Harvard. Louis was, Holmes recalled, "a tall, rather spare, dignified personage, of serene and grave aspect,"[3] a man who "taught us who followed him the love of truth, the habit of passionless listening to the teachings of nature." But he was not, in any conventional sense, an inspiring teacher: "he was not a showy, or eloquent, or, I should say, a very generally popular man, though the favorite, almost the idol, of many students, especially Genevese and Bostonians."[4]

At the same time, Holmes's language of moral integrity—what he means to get at in speaking of his teacher's "love of truth"—immediately points to the basis of Louis's appeal to American students during this period of medical history. The same note shows up again and again in reminiscences by Louis's American disciples, a sign that their teacher had become for them the very symbol not simply of originality or brilliance in medical research, but of disinterested inquiry itself, or what in a more innocent age could be called the pursuit of truth for its own sake. Louis was, observes Howard Payson Arnold in his memoir of Mason Warren, "the most careful, impartial, and honest observer that his profession had yet known. . . . Eager for the truth, and aware that of all dangers a fallacious certainty is the greatest, he was always seeking for more light. He was quick to detect error in any guise, however plausible, and dreaded only that darkness which is the offspring of bigotry and ignorance."[5] Yet the aura of moral and intellectual integrity that surrounded Louis in the eyes of his American students was, as Bowditch and Holmes also make clear, something wholly unperceived by French medical students.

The reason why this should be so is amply provided, I think, in John Harley Warner's *Against the Spirit of System*, a study of the American doctors who studied in Paris in the earlier part of the nineteenth century. For the story Warner tells concerns the relentless pressures of the marketplace in a nation so new that institutions, customs, and traditions provide no countervailing influence, a struggle for medical authority in a world where market relations and numerical democracy are the only recognized sources of social legitimacy. Warner's accomplishment is thus to have set nineteenth century American medicine in the context of a theme that goes back to Tocqueville's *Democracy in America*, the idea that Jacksonian democracy, along with its political triumph, had unleashed the forces of a raw economic individualism that would come to dominate every aspect of American culture. "The love of wealth," Tocqueville reported to his European readers, is "to be traced, as either a principal or an accessory motive, at the bottom of all the Americans do; . . . The perpetual recurrence of the same passion is monotonous. The peculiar methods by which this passion seeks its own gratification are not less so."[6]

The dilemma of the American physician, in this context, was to discover a genuine source of medical authority in a society, to borrow Quentin Anderson's memorable phrase, "imaginatively dominated by money and the process of exchange."[7] Consider, for instance, the career of Holmes's friend James Jackson, Jr., whom Dr. Louis would come to see not simply as his most promising student, but almost as a son. His father, James Jackson, Sr., was a Harvard professor and one of America's leading physicians. After the untimely death of his son at the age of 24, the senior Jackson would become a principal spokesman for Louis's doctrines in America. During young Jackson's lifetime, the only point of contention that would arise between the two older physicians involved the issue of pure medical research. Their exchange of views on the topic began when Louis wrote the senior Jackson to tell him that his son had an exceptional talent for clinical observation. He urged that the young man be allowed, after returning to Boston, to devote several more years to the same sort of research he has been carrying out with Louis at La Pitié:

> Let us suppose that he should pass four more years without engaging in the practice of medicine, what a mass of positive knowledge will he have acquired! How many important results will he have been able to publish to the world during that period! After that he must necessarily become one of the bright lights of his country. Others will resort to him for instruction, and he will be able to impart it with distinguished honor to himself. If all these things be duly weighed, it will appear that he will soon redeem the four years, which men of superficial views will believe him to have lost.[8]

Thus begins an exchange in which Louis may be heard as spokesman for a Paris medicine that, in an older European civilization, has always been able simply to assume its exemption from the operations of the marketplace. In the distant background of Louis's proposal to Jackson, Sr., lies, for instance, the medieval guild concept of a trade or profession, one originally designed as much to protect guild members from unfair or unscrupulous competition as to enforce standards of quality or competence. From the Renaissance onward, with Galenic doctrine making a knowledge of Latin and Greek a precondition of medical study, this would give way to university training and certification by diploma—the lengthy process that at Oxford, as we saw in an earlier chapter, would produce a doctor of medicine only after fourteen years of study. In eighteenth-century England, as Lester King has pointed out, the Royal College of Physicians "was in essence a feudal guild, or at least a direct lineal descendant thereof, an example of that system which gave a protected favored position to its members in return for specified services."[9] In eighteenth-century France, where the ancient and privileged Medical Faculty had long since succumbed to what Ackerknecht calls "the dry rot of the *ancien régime*,"[10] the Royal Society of Medicine was founded by a group of progressive physicians in 1776 with a similar purpose in mind.

The French Revolution had swept away the medical training of the *ancien régime*, which French medical reformers described as a dreary round of Latin lectures delivered by a superannuated faculty selected on a principle of rotation. As we have seen, it did so in favor of a system meant to recognize knowledge and competence as the sole basis of medical authority. As American students instantly and appreciatively understood, the effect of the *concours* was to put rich and poor on an equal footing—this is, once again, the story of Velpeau as a parable of sheer talent and industry[11]—while ensuring the selection of the most gifted candidates. Thus, for instance, the lament of a dispirited Augustus Gardner, who has just learned that twenty hospital positions in his own New York City are to be filled by political appointment. Not a single position has been set aside for a candidate who "shows himself to be really the first man in the particular department of the profession to which he is elected."[12] The final triumph of the *concours* system was then to set the most gifted Paris physicians outside the marketplace. The salaries of those whom *Paris médicale* called the princes of medicine—the Dupuytrens, Chomels, Andrals—were paid by the state. And their lectures, as William Gibson wonderingly remarked in 1839, "were paid for by government, and *gratuitous*, as respected the student."[13]

The elder Jackson must have felt, as he sat down to answer Louis's letter, an almost anthropological sense of strangeness, as though he had somehow had thrust upon him the unhappy burden of explaining American peculiarities to someone dwelling within an utterly different system of values and beliefs. Nonetheless, he does his best to explain to Louis that his proposal is not a simple question of paternal permission granted or withheld, but of implacable social conditions beyond the control of any individual. In the United States, he tells his Parisian colleague, "every young man engages as soon as he can in the business of life. . . . Most of our physicians go into business after three years of study; some, by visiting foreign schools, protract the period of study to five or six years. If now, after this longer period, one should at the present day, spend four or five years longer in the acquisition of professional knowledge, he would be regarded as a singular being, governed by a peculiar taste; and it would probably be thought that he would never be fit for the active business of life."[14]

In the same way, Jackson's letter to Dr. Louis echoes those passages in Tocqueville that try to get across to European readers a sense of the strangeness of a country in which market relations are the sole basis of social reality. So, for instance, Tocqueville: "Americans are constantly driven to engage in commerce and industry. . . . Even the region they inhabit urge[s] them irresistibly in this direction. Their present condition . . . is that of an almost exclusively manufacturing and commercial association, placed in the midst of a new and boundless country, which their principle object is to explore for purposes of profit."[15] Similarly, Jackson, Sr., doing his best to explain to Dr. Louis why granting his son a period of pure research would deny him any future success as a physician: "In this country his course would have been so singular, as in a measure to separate him from other men. We are a business doing people. We are new. We have, as it were, but just landed on these uncultivated shores; there is a vast deal to be done; and he who will not be doing, must be set down as a drone. If he is a drone in appearance only and not in fact, it will require a long time to prove it so, when his character has once been fixed in the public mind."[16]

James Jackson, Jr., would come down with a grievous illness and die within two years of his return to America in 1833. In Boston, his death was understood as a symbolic event. In the passing of the younger Jackson, said a notice in the *Boston Daily Advertiser*, "a thousand expectations are shattered. We have no right to use the language of private and exclusive sorrow. He belonged to the public."[17] There is in such eulogies the unmistakable implication of a vanished ideal. No one who knew Jackson's allegiance to Louis and Paris medicine was unaware of what that ideal was. To the public beyond his circle of acquaintance, it was made clear in the letters from Paris included in the *Memoir* published by his father shortly after his son's death. "In very truth," the younger Jackson had said in one of these, "I look forward with fear and trembling to the day when I *must* employ my time to earn money, instead of to learn truth. . . . Persuaded as I am that there is very much in the exercise of our profession, that develops and satisfies the affections,—that delights the moral man—yet I must acknowledge that, had circumstances favored it, I should have been pleased to pass at least eight or ten years in the study of the sciences of pathology and therapeutics, in the hopes of establishing some important truths."[18]

It is the voice of Paris medicine. "If our profession ever vindicates its legitimate claim to the appellation of liberal," Elisha Bartlett had written in 1831, shortly after his own homecoming from Paris, "it must be cultivated with some other than the single aim of obtaining patients for the sole purpose of getting for services rendered an equivalent in fees."[19] The *Memoir of James Jackson, Jr.* written by his father would keep alive in the Boston medical community an ideal that might otherwise have been thought to have gone to the grave with the son. For the *Memoir* served not only as a repository of values that seemed elsewhere to have been obliterated by the economic individualism associated with Jacksonian democracy—an America consisting, as Tocqueville put it, of "an innumerable multitude of men, all equal and alike, incessantly endeavoring to procure the petty and paltry pleasures with which they glut their lives"[20]—but, especially in Boston, would preserve the younger Jackson's relationship to Louis as an emblem of the pursuit of truth for its own sake.[21] Half a century later, Holmes would go out of his way to recall for his own students the memory of James Jackson, Jr., as "a young man whose early death was a calamity to the profession of which he promised to be a chief ornament."[22]

In the years following the younger Jackson's death, the distinguishing mark of Boston clinical practice would be a resistance to the forces of the American marketplace. Appropriately enough, it was the next round of P. C. A. Louis's researches, published in 1835 as *Recherches sur les effets de la saignée dans quelques maladies inflammatoires*, that would provide the basis of resistance. For the earlier work that had given Louis an international reputation—and, in the process, given the coup de grâce to Broussais's system of "physiological medicine"—was his *Researches on Phthisis*, which had said next to nothing about the implications of his numerical method for judging therapeutic regimens. The new work, immediately translated and published in Boston as *Researches on the Effects of Bloodletting* (1836) with a foreword by James Jackson, Sr., took on the issue in direct terms. What Louis did, we recall Holmes saying in his lecture to his last anatomy class, was to show "by a strict analysis of numerous cases that bleeding did not strangle,—*jugulate* was the word then used,—acute diseases. . . . This was not a reform,—it was a revolution."[23]

The use of phlebotomy in disease was, as we have seen, as old as Galenic medicine, whose theory of humoral imbalance—*plethora* was the specific condition that demanded bloodletting by venesection, cupping, or the application of leeches—was the most obvious sign of the physician's competence and authority. In the American colonies before the Revolution, British-trained physicians would often remark that their colonial counterparts carried bloodletting and other "heroic" measures to excess, no doubt because in the absence of such certifying badges as university diplomas or membership in the Royal College of Physicians, the therapy itself amounted to a form of certification. "In general the physical practice in our colonies is so perniciously bad," William Douglass would remark in 1750, "that, excepting in surgery and some very acute cases, it is better to let nature, under a proper regimen, take her course than to trust to the honesty and sagacity of the practitioner. . . . When I first arrived in New England . . . a most facetious practitioner . . . told me their practice was very uniform: bleeding, vomiting, blistering, purging, anodynes, etc. If the illness continued, there was *repetendi*, and finally *murderandi*; nature was never to be consulted or allowed to have any concern in the affair."[24]

In the period following the American Revolution, however, these therapies would be given the stamp of American democracy by Benjamin Rush, the Jeffersonian physician whose doctrines still dominated American medicine when Bostonians like Oliver Wendell Holmes were studying in Paris.[25] Nor was the relationship between Jeffersonian democratic ideology and Rush's theories lost on those who would lead the resistance to marketplace medicine. Thus, for instance, Holmes himself in "Currents and Counter-Currents in Medical Science": "who can fail to recognize that Benjamin Rush, the most conspicuous of American physicians, was the intellectual offspring of the movement which produced the Revolution? 'The same hand,' says one of his biographers, 'which subscribed the declaration of the political independence of these States, accomplished their emancipation from medical systems formed in foreign countries'."[26] "Dr. Rush thought and said," remarks Holmes in the same essay, "that there were twenty times more intellect and a hundred times more knowledge in the country in 1799 than before the Revolution. His own mind was in a perpetual state of exaltation produced by . . . the quickened life of the time in which he lived."[27]

The relationship between politics and medicine intuited by Holmes at such moments had to do, specifically, with the role of systems, meaning abstract doctrines presented in terms of an ideal rationality. In politics, this involved the sort of speculative tinkering with traditional or customary social arrangements denounced by Burke in *Reflections on the Revolution in France*, the point of his mocking references to "metaphysical doctors of the rights of man." For both Thomas Jefferson and Benjamin Rush, whose deep sympathies with revolutionary France would survive even the Reign of Terror, it was precisely the abstract doctrines of liberty and equality that gave the French Revolution its kinship with their own.[28] In medicine, the epiphany that produced Rush's system would come to him during the Philadelphia yellow fever epidemic of 1793, when he recollected some old medical manuscripts about an earlier epidemic. They were the basis of his revelation that the cure for this disease, and all others, was to remove excess stimulus from the system. "Never before did I experience such sublime joy," he would later recall, "as I now felt in contemplating the success of my remedies. It repaid me for all the toils and studies of my life."[29]

The basis for Rush's moment of illumination had doubtless been laid by his teacher William Cullen, who had theorized that fever, though present in numerous diseases, was due to spasm in the capillary vessels. Yet what Cullen had failed to see, and what Rush was now permitted to see in a moment of sudden clarity, was that fever was the seat of disease: "All ordinary fever being seated in the blood vessels, it follows . . . that all those local affections we call pleurisy, angina, phrenitis, internal dropsy of the brain, pulmonary consumption, and inflammation of the liver, stomach, bowels, and limbs, are symptoms only of an original and primary disease in the sanguiferous system."[30] The origins of Rush's theory, as of John Brown's theory of excitability or Broussais's doctrine of gastrointestinal inflammation, may no doubt be traced to the iatrophysics of Boerhaave, which taught that bodily heat was produced by the mechanical friction of blood moving through the circulatory system. Yet Rush's "capillary tension" had the enormous advantage of being a medical theory that could be easily grasped by ordinary citizens in a democratic republic.

In Rush's case, in short, the relation between political ideology and medical theory is to be sought not in the therapeutic practice for which he is primarily known among historians of medicine—as we have seen, this was merely an intensification of a regimen already well-established in colonial America—but in the way he set about justifying it to a citizenry entitled to know precisely why it was being bled and purged and blistered by its physicians. This is the basis, for instance, for Rush's open contempt for the nosological systems of the Old World, such as Pinel's elaborate classification of fevers. For the multiplication of diseases, Rush would grandly proclaim, is "as repugnant to truth in medicine, as polytheism is to truth in religion. The physician who considers every different affection of the different systems of the body . . . as distinct diseases when they arise from one cause, resembles the Indian or African savage, who considers water, dew, ice, frost and snow as distinct essences."[31] So it is that fever must be viewed as a single entity, as fire is a single entity "whether it be produced by friction, percussion, electricity, fermentation, or by a piece of wood or coal in a state of inflammation."[32]

Given conditions in the medical marketplace of the early American republic, the great advantage of Rush's theory was that it justifed what physicians had already been doing under the rubric of antiphlogistic treatment: the supposed reduction of inflammatory symptoms by variations on the older Galenic regimen of bleeding, purging, and blistering. Some elements were simply holdovers from the older humoral pathology, as with the placing of setons, or ligatures that, becoming infected, set up a counterirritation meant to draw blood away from the primary seat of inflammation. In the same way, the giving of emetics and cathartics—substances that made the patient vomit or violently move the bowels—was meant to accelerate the actions of the body as a system already attempting to purge itself of a plethoric excess. The major impact of Rush's theory was to justify pursuing these same measures to a "heroic" level. "The term *heroic*," explains John Harley Warner, "reflected the belief that aggressive intervention was often called for to effect the therapeutic lowering. . . . Heroic depletion was brought about by such drugs as cathartics (calomel, corrosive sublimate, jalap), emetics (tartar emetic, ipecacuanha), and counterirritants (blisters), by low diet, and by drawing blood."[33]

Underlying the system of heroic intervention was the notion that nature, when permitted to pursue her own course, led invariably to a deleterious state of affairs. Again, the political overtones of Rush's animus against "nature" are unmistakable. Just as a long, slow, unsupervised accretion of custom and tradition had led to ministerial tyranny in Britain and the *ancien régime* in France, the unimpeded course of nature in disease could lead only to debility and death. "It is impossible to calculate the mischief which Hippocrates has done," said Rush in a pronouncement quoted by Holmes in "Currents and Counter-Currents", "by first marking Nature with his name and afterwards letting her loose upon sick people. Millions have perished by her hands in all ages and countries."[34] "In all violent diseases," Rush told his students, "nature is like a drunken man reeling to & fro & occasionally stumbling against a door with so much violence as to break it through. Always treat nature in a sick room as you would a noisy dog or cat; drive her out at the door & lock it upon her."[35] The medical students who went forth from Rush's classes at the University of Pennsylvania knew precisely what means were to be taken to expel Nature when they met her in the sickroom of a grievously ill patient.

The most dramatic of these was bloodletting. For the same theory that posited fever as the seat of all disease, and a disorder of the blood vessels—what we have heard Rush call "an original and primary disease in the sanguiferous system"—as the cause of fever, taught that the single most powerful remedy available to the physician was venesection. This, in Rush's own view, was the major advantage of his own system over those that imagined diseases to be separate entities demanding separate modes of treatment: "We will suppose the Doctor to have a house containing 100 rooms, each having a different Lock; of course he must have an equal number of different Keys to open them—now I am capable of entering every apartment in my House with the assistance of a Single Key."[36] Against objections that excessive bloodletting might weaken the patient as much or more than the disease it was supposed to cure, Rush marshaled his own theory of capillary tension: up to four-fifths of the blood could be removed from the body, he maintained, without danger to the patient: "'Tis a very hard Matter to bleed a Patient to Death, provided the Blood be not drawn from a Vital part."[37]

In the Boston medical community, where the influence of Paris medicine was most pronounced, and where the appearance of Louis's *Researches on Bloodletting* would bring about an almost immediate reaction against massive bloodletting, the practice of bleeding patients to death would have all but faded away by midcentury. But elsewhere in the United States, where a resort to heroic measures would persist as the most visible sign of the physician's authority and competence, Rush's single key to the many-doored house of disease never lost its status as a favorite remedy. Consider, for instance, the way the wife of Salmon P. Chase, Lincoln's Secretary of the Treasury, was treated for puerperal fever by her physicians:

> Dr. Colby, thinking she had been bled as much as her constitution would bear, . . . arrested the flow of blood. Dr. Drake was much dissatisfied, and insisted upon a more copious bleeding. The bandage was accordingly removed, and more blood taken. It was then replaced. Dr. Drake still remained unsatisfied, urging that it was necessary to bleed to fainting. . . . Kitty was told that the doctors thought of bleeding her again, and was asked if she was willing. She said "Yes, anything." She was then raised up in bed, and twenty ounces of blood were taken from her. The effect on the pulse was the exact contrary of what was anticipated. It became more frequent and more feeble. . . . The [patient's] father came into [her] room exclaiming, "Thank God, my child, the doctors say there is hope." She said nothing. All hope had vanished. . . . Dr. Drake felt her pulse, and said she was dead.[38]

Even in the last quarter of the nineteenth century, long after the "Parisian" arguments of physicians like Jacob Bigelow and Oliver Wendell Holmes had penetrated to medical colleges in remote states, and after movements like Thomsonian botanical medicine had mounted a popular resistance to bloodletting, venesection would in some areas remain the outward sign of medical authority. "I was acquainted with a neighboring physician who proposed to cure and did cure common intermittent [i.e., malaria] by blood-letting alone," recalled G. S. B. Hempstead in 1878. "He bled the patient till he was too weak to shake, and then the disease and the patient went off together. I mention this to show the recklessness of doctors in the use of the lancet, and of patients in submitting to it."[39] Even in Boston, the center of the resistance to heroic measures in therapy, it would never die out completely. "A fortnight ago," reports a bemused Holmes in a talk delivered to medical students in 1867, "I found myself in the cars with one of the most sensible and esteemed practitioners in New England. He took out his wallet and showed me two lancets, which he carried with him; he had never given up their use."[40]

The other heroic measure licensed by Rush's single-disease theory was the use of violent emetics and cathartics, again a modern adaptation of remedies used in the older Galenic or humoral medicine. The main innovation was the use of mineral substances such as mercury and antimony—represented in the materia medica of the ordinary physician by calomel, a mercury preparation, and tartar emetic, an antimony compound—in place of the herbal and vegetable remedies used by ancient and medieval physicians. In the case of mercury, however, the argument against its use was not nearly as conclusive as that against bloodletting. For mercury, in this instance best regarded as an early form of chemotherapy, was the only known cure for syphilis, a disease more terrible in its terminal stages than the most noxious of remedies. Holmes, an articulate opponent of the widespread use of calomel—the mercury it contained, he argued, was "alien to the system, and eminently disturbing in its influence"—was compelled to admit that the case against its use was complicated by its undoubted power against syphilis. "Its efficacy in certain forms of specific disease," as he would decorously phrase it, "is acknowledged by all but the most skeptical of theorists."[41]

Holmes's source for this opinion was his Paris teacher Philippe Ricord, then recognized as the world's leading authority on venereal diseases.[42] As late as the beginning of the twentieth century, the efficacy of mercuric rubs as a specific against syphilis was unreservedly maintained by the pioneer syphilologist John H. Stokes, even as Ehrlich's Salvarsan was arriving on the scene to usher in a new era of treatment: "In eight years of systematic use of the inunction as interim treatment by some ten thousand patients who have taken an aggregate of hundreds of thousands of rubs I can personally testify to this really extraordinary factor of safety combined with therapeutic effectiveness." Yet Stokes himself confessed that mercury "has always been a storm center of therapeutics,"[43] which is what Holmes had in mind, in the essay just quoted, in going on to observe that "there is no telling what evils have arisen from the abuse of this mineral."[44] In 1858, Nathan Knepfler described the terrible effects of mercury treatment even when warranted by syphilis:

The mouth feels unusually hot . . . ; the gums are swollen, red, and tender, ulcers make their appearance and spread in all directions; the saliva is thick and stringy, and has that peculiar, offensive odor characteristic of mercurial disease; the tongue is swollen and stiff, and there is some fever. . . . The disease progressing, it destroys every part that it touches, until the lips, the cheeks, and even the bones have been eaten away. . . . The teeth . . . become loose and rot, perhaps fall out; or worse still, the upper and lower jaw-bones exfoliate and rot out sometimes . . . and the poor object lingers out a doleful existence during life. . . . This happens when mercury performs a *cure!*[45]

The campaign waged by Holmes and other Boston physicians against calomel would be based on the argument that, given such terrible effects, there was no justification for using mercury in cases where its therapeutic value had not been proven. This was the basis, for instance, of the plea made by John Collins Warren, father of Mason, against all medicines that endangered the safety of the patient: "let me invite the experienced and conscientious practitioner to turn his eyes back to the mercurial practice, and witness the sloughing gums, necrosed jaws, inveterate ulcers, and ruined constitutions, produced by mercury, and then say whether he can bring forward a well-observed series of satisfactory cures to counterbalance these evils."[46] Holmes would be making much the same point in observing that even horticulturists know that some substances are deadly to plants. "There is a presumption against putting lead or arsenic into the human body," he argued, "as against putting them into plants, because they do not belong there. . . . The same is true of mercury and silver. What becomes of these alien substances after they get into the system we cannot always tell."[47]

Yet the use of calomel and other violent purgatives would persist as an outward sign of medical competence. Benjamin Rush was especially known for prescribing jalap, a purgative the harshness of whose action, as William Rothstein remarks, "can best be judged by recognizing that it was mixed with calomel to make it more palatable."[48] Rush had instituted the practice of mixing calomel and jalap—ten grains of each, reported by one of Rush's students to be a dose considered "perfectly enormous"—during the Philadelphia yellow fever epidemic of 1793. Here again, Holmes glimpsed a relation to Jeffersonian ideology. Rush, he wryly observed, "could not help feeling as if Nature had been a good deal shaken by the Declaration of Independence, and that American art was getting to be rather too much for her. . . . How could a people which . . . contrived the Bowie-knife and the revolver, which has chewed the juice out of all the superlatives in the language in Fourth of July orations . . . be content with any but 'heroic' practice? What wonder that the stars and stripes wave over doses of ninety grains of sulphate of quinine, and that the American eagle screams with delight to see three drachms of calomel given at a single mouthful."[49]

This is the background against which P. C. A. Louis's *Recherches sur les effets de la saignée* would appear in English translation in Boston in 1836, only a year after its original publication in Paris. It catalyzed a strong reaction against heroic practice in the Boston medical community, the origins of which may be traced to James Jackson, Jr.'s return from Paris in 1833. For though Louis was known in America mainly for his 1825 treatise on phthisis, the young Jackson had in Paris gotten a first-hand acquaintance with his teacher's work on the effects of bloodletting in serious diseases, especially pneumonia. The first stirrings of that therapeutic skepticism that would become the hallmark of Boston medicine appear in the younger Jackson's letters to his father, usually to make the point that nothing in the current teaching of therapy meets the standard of certainty established by Paris anatomico-pathological research. "Do I believe that bleeding *arrests* inflammation, as I believe that a certain combination of symptoms indicates such and such a lesion? Is not the last proved by numerous demonstrations? Have I ever seen *one* instance of what the books talk so easily of as to the first?"[50]

After the appearance of Louis's *Researches on Bloodletting*, the letters from young Jackson preserved in his father's *Memoir* could be taken in Boston as a virtual manifesto against heroic practice, and, even more importantly, against the monstrous spectacle of ignorance masquerading as medical knowledge. "Just reflect for a moment," he entreats his father, "of what materials our therapeutic literature consists: almost without exception, chosen cases to prove the efficacy of such and such remedies. Is this the way to proceed? Suppose the chemist went to his laboratory *hoping* to find oxygen in *everything*, and made known to the public only those cases in which he found it; would his science advance?"[51] Or, similarly—one hears already the voices of Jacob Bigelow and Oliver Wendell Holmes advancing nearly identical arguments—how, when the physician has treated a disease, does he know that it was his remedy that worked? "When life is threatened, do we very often save it? When a disease is destined by *nature* to be long, do we very often materially diminish it? . . . I must acknowledge that, what I have seen here of disease and its issues, has rather inclined me to believe that I *individually* overvalued the utility of certain modes of treatment in America."[52]

The message sent by Louis's *Researches on Bloodletting*, in short, carried through to every aspect of American medical practice. If bleeding killed people as often as it cured them—or, nearly as bad, "cured" them only in the sense that they got well despite the bloodletting—were there not grounds to suspect that massive doses of calomel and jalap, so obviously violent in their effects on the patient, were also hastening the death of those who had sent for the doctor in hopes of being made well? The answer, in the opinion of disciples like James Jackson, Jr., but also, eventually, in that of virtually every leading member of the Boston medical community, could only be provided by Louis's numerical method, an early version of what we should now call a controlled experiment or clinical trial. Mason Warren, who, as we recall, had gotten permission from his father to spend an additional year in Paris solely to study with Louis, gives a detailed description of how the system worked. What Mason calls *peripneumons* are what we should now call cases of pneumonia:

His method is this: he takes, for instance in Peripneumons, 40 patients; half are bled before the 4th day and half after. In those bled before, the disease lasted 16 days; in those after, 20. He observes in the same way the effect of other means of treatment. He analyses the different symptoms of the disease. He finds, for instance, how long the [illegible] expectoration lasts in patients affected with Inflammation of the superior lobe and how long in those of the inferior lobe; how long the *crépitant râle* endured in the former and in the latter and discovers that with the change in expectoration there is a change in the *râle*. . . . By these means of [numbering] the cases he arrives at results which are certain and which often go entirely against what has been from ages admitted as true.[53]

The origins of Louis's numerical system lay, as Ackerknecht points out, in the nosological classifications of Pinel. For Pinel had been not only a physician but a mathematician who resorted to statistical method—"*le calcul des probabilités*"—whenever possible.[54] In more general terms, it reflected what Holmes once called "the observing and computing mind of the nineteenth century": "The two dominant words of our time are *law* and *average*, both pointing to the uniformity of the order of being in which we live. Statistics have tabulated everything. . . . Analysis and classification have been at work upon all tangible and visible objects."[55] Yet statistics as such were not, for Louis's Boston readers, the crucial feature of his system. That feature was, rather, as James Jackson, Sr., would point out, that Louis's method renounced speculative hypotheses in favor of verifiable results: "Unlike the systems, which are always spoken of in the history of medicine, as successively rising with splendor and falling into oblivion, the principles published by the founder of the numerical system are not an artificial network, where the cutting of one thread may cause the whole to drop away; these principles may be . . . enlarged, limited, and modified, and yet the system may be maintained."[56]

The silent revolution brought about by Louis's *Researches on Bloodletting* was to transform the way Boston physicians, along with a few scattered souls outside New England, viewed medical controversy itself. Elsewhere such controversy would remain, as it had been since the days of Galen and Celsus, primarily a contest of personal authority, with dominant personalities like Benjamin Rush or François Joseph Victor Broussais arguing for some system with which their own name was popularly associated. In Boston, after the lessons of James Jackson, Sr.'s *Memoir* of his son and the translations of Louis's major works had sunk in, it would instead be understood as a contest between speculative systems and the laws of nature: a dispute in which an honorable controversialist ought simply to set out results or conclusions that could be verified by other researchers and then step aside, leaving his opponents to deal with a physical reality oblivious to rhetoric or persuasion. As we shall see, Holmes's specialized treatise on puerperal fever, marking a crucial stage in his development as author of *The Autocrat of the Breakfast Table* and other purely literary works, would carry this new mode of controversy through to a triumphant conclusion.

In the immediate background of Holmes's *The Contagiousness of Puerperal Fever* stands Louis's *Examen de l'éxamen de M. Broussais relativement à la phthisie et à l'affection typoïde*, a response to Broussais published in Paris in 1834, when Holmes was his student at La Pitié. Broussais, unwilling to let Laennec's death lay to rest his ongoing feud with *l'école de La Charité*, had in the latest edition of his *Examen* turned against Louis, attacking, in particular, his researches on phthisis and typhoid fever. Broussais's attack was, as usual, brutal in its *ad hominem* violence, its deliberate misrepresentation of the works it purported to be objectively examining, and its self-aggrandizing promotion of his own system of *la médecine physiologique*. It portrayed Louis as an assiduous, subservient, even sycophantic pupil of Laennec, and as Laennec's anointed successor in the study of tuberculosis through diagnosis by percussion and auscultation. In specific terms, it presented Broussais's own pathological findings as evidence against the "laws"—in Louis's usage, the term for statistically reliable correlations—governing the occurrence of tubercles as lesions in various states and stages of disease.

The tone of Louis's *Examen de l'éxamen* is more tempered and aggrieved than openly outraged, though one senses a current of molten anger running just beneath the surface. To Broussais's charge that he is Laennec's subservient pupil, his answer is simple: he only saw Laennec twice in his life. He never attended Laennec's classes or clinical rounds. After returning from a period of medical practice in Russia, he had attended the lessons of only one professor of internal pathology—namely, M. Broussais himself.[57] Yet Louis's most telling response is to Broussais's grand pronouncement that his researches have added nothing to "pathological, therapeutic, or hygienic knowledge, let alone to our knowledge of physiology." This is, Louis quietly remarks, an odd sort of reproach,

one that I must admit I accept rather as a eulogy, for it gives a very precise idea of the spirit in which I have devoted myself to my research. In fact, I was trying to make as sure then as I do today that I never set anything out as a result that does not derive directly from my observed facts, that I make every attempt to avoid presenting my "approach," or my opinions in pathology, therapy, or hygiene, as truths. For in medicine what are normally called opinions, or insights, or approaches, belong, properly speaking, to scientific fantasy. This is perhaps why, in reading the work of M. Broussais, I have so often felt a sharp regret that they are so teeming with theories, opinions, and physiological, pathological, and therapeutic insights that are not anchored in the results of rigorous, and therefore truly useful, observation.[58]

This is the voice of the Louis whose *Researches on Phthisis* and later work on typhoid fever would, by freeing medicine from merely speculative theories, establish a ground of sound empirical evidence as the only valid basis for the study of disease. Until Louis perfected the numerical system, Holmes would say, "the history of practical medicine had been the story of the Danaides. 'Experience' had been, from time immemorial, pouring its flowing treasures into buckets full of holes. At the existing rate of supply and leakage they would never be filled: nothing would ever be settled in medicine."[59] The effect of Louis's *Researches on Bloodletting*, on the other hand, would be to suggest to his Boston readers, along with a new perspective on the subject of therapeutics, nothing less than an entirely new conception of medical authority and competence. This is the direction in which James Jackson, Jr., had already been moving in those letters from Paris in which he registered a skepticism not simply about phlebotomy, but about every remedy conventionally listed in the American materia medica. After studying with Louis, his father told readers of his *Memoir of James Jackson, Jr.*, his son could not bring himself to "feel a reliance, in respect to the influence of medicine, on the experience of men, who could not tell what would be the result of a disease without the use of remedies."[60]

After his son's death, the senior Jackson would be among the leading spokesmen in America for the *méthode expectante*, or conscious policy of doing nothing to hinder the body in its natural efforts to overcome disease. "I would advise a young physician to adopt the *expectant* mode of treatment recommended by some physicians of France," he goes on to say in the *Memoir*, "rather than to employ on every occasion the heroic remedies of some of our countrymen. The profuse use of these remedies, . . . too often witnessed among us, cannot be too openly, nor too loudly reprobated. These errors are disgraceful to our profession."[61] Yet he would always make clear that this was not mere therapeutic nihilism, but allegiance to the same empirical standards that had produced such incontestably reliable results in Paris anatomico-pathological medicine:

> Let M. Louis, or men like him, test the effect of remedies in the same spirit, with which he has pursued his pathological researches. Having determined the average duration, fatality, &c. of typhus, for example, by an observation of a sufficient number of cases through a series of years, such cases not having been actively treated, let him then employ in the same disease those which have been thought useful. One physician extols the advantages of bleeding; another commends antimonials employed in the first days of the disease, in emetic doses, and for a few days afterwards in doses just short of nauseating. . . . Let each mode of treatment have its

fair trial; and let the results be compared with each other, and with similar cases, treated at the same time upon the expectant method.[62]

Dr. Jackson's voice would almost immediately be joined by that of John Collins Warren, and within a short time by those of such younger physicians as Elisha Bartlett and Mason Warren and Oliver Wendell Holmes, until the *méthode expectante* had become the virtual hallmark of Boston medicine.[63] In American medicine generally, the very phrase *médecine expectante* signaled nervous awareness of a therapeutic hiatus that would last well into the early twentieth century, long after Paris anatomico-pathological research, the cell biology of Virchow and the German school, and the germ theory of Louis Pasteur had brought about tremendous advances in understanding the etiology and physiology of disease.[64] The idea of a physician who could do nothing to cure illness, and who used a French phrase to declare his helplessness, seemed like an open confession of professional failure to those raised on Rush's exhortations to heroic intervention. Yet in Boston it would signal something else as well: a conscious determination to resist the forces of the marketplace in American medicine. It was this resistance that demanded, as its rationale, a new conception of medical competence and authority.

That rationale was provided in Jacob Bigelow's "On Self-Limited Diseases," given as a talk at the annual meeting of the Massachusetts Medical Society in 1835. Bigelow's discourse, Holmes could still maintain in a Lowell Institute lecture given over thirty years later, was "an address which can be read in a single hour, but the influence of which will be felt for a century."[65] In Holmes's final lecture to his Harvard anatomy class, he would again recall Bigelow's talk, this time as giving systematic expression to the teachings of P. C. A. Louis in his rounds at La Pitié: "One thing, at any rate, we did learn in the wards of Louis. We learned that a very large proportion of diseases get well of themselves, without any specific medication,—the great fact formulated, enforced, and popularized by Dr. Jacob Bigelow in the Discourse referred to. We *un*learned the habit of drugging for its own sake."[66] Yet Bigelow's address, written in the somewhat ungainly prose of a man more at home in the examining room than on a lecture platform, was much more than a mere attempt to popularize the therapeutic skepticism authorized by Louis's *Researches on Bloodletting*. It was Boston's declaration of independence from a medical marketplace driven by the new economic individualism associated with Jacksonian democracy.

The overall tone of Bigelow's discourse is commonsensical, meant to appeal to the experience of any physician who has treated ordinary illness, or even of any parent who has seen a child through the ordinary course of childhood diseases. Every mother knows, for instance, that childhood cases of chickenpox and measles run their course and get well by themselves. A new mother wanting to know what to expect when her child comes down with mumps will simply go and ask more experienced women in the neighborhood. In the same way, every physician knows that there is a tremendous variability in the onset and severity of contagious diseases. In an epidemic of smallpox or scarlet fever, some people will become grievously ill and die, some will become moderately ill and recover, and others still have cases of the disease so mild as scarcely to cause them inconvenience. Just as important is that many of these diseases, when the patient has caught them and recovered, bestow a lifelong immunity on the patient thereafter. This had been, as anyone in Bigelow's audience could be counted upon to know, the basis of inoculation for smallpox when introduced into England by Lady Mary Wortley Montague, and into New England by Cotton Mather.[67] It was the basis of vaccination as practiced after Jenner's discovery that cowpox acted as an immunizing agent.

Yet it had taken Paris medicine to show physicians who had not surrendered to a blind allegiance to heroic practice that a great many diseases are precisely like the measles and chickenpox of childhood, separate entities that, having gained entry to the body as a physical system, run a course impervious to the commonly used therapeutic measures. This is something that Holmes himself saw clearly almost as soon as he returned from Paris. "One half the opposition which the numerical system of Louis has met with, as applied to the results of treatment," he would later observe, "has been owing to the fact that it showed the movements of disease to be far more independent of the kind of practice pursued than was agreeable to the pride of those whose self-confidence it abated."[68] This was the context in which Bigelow's mere definition of a self-limited disease would have been instantly grasped by any American physician as a grave threat to prevailing notions of therapeutic practice. For by such a disease Bigelow meant "one which, after it has obtained foothold in the system, cannot, in the present state of our knowledge, be eradicated, or abridged, by art,—but to which there is due a certain succession of processes, to be completed in a certain time."[69]

At just this point, the authority of Paris medicine becomes crucial to Bigelow's case. For he is addressing a Boston audience, already aware of P. C. A. Louis's reputation for uncompromising moral and intellectual integrity. Thus Bigelow's simple proposal that Louis's system be applied to American therapeutics carries enormous preemptive weight: "The *numerical* method employed by Louis, . . . and now adopted by his most distinguished contemporaries in France, affords the means of as near an approach to certainty on this head, as the subject itself admits."[70] As importantly, he is able to invoke Louis and Andral in direct support of his own concept of self-limited diseases. For Louis has already stated that typhoid fever, once established in the system, cannot be altered by therapy. Bigelow, no doubt to drive home the point that a knowledge of Paris medicine is needed to grasp the truth on this subject, cites both Louis and Andral in the original. Louis: "L'experience ayant montré, que l'affection typhoide bien caractérisée, n'est pas susceptible d'etre jugulée, ce qui n'est guere moins vrai, d'ailleurs . . . de la peripneumonie et des autres maladies inflammatoires." Andral: "Quelles que soient les méthodes employées, il est un certain nombre de cas òu, sans que ces methodes y prennent part, la nature conduit la maladie à une termination heureuse ou funeste."[71]

A question then arises which, when it is first introduced, Bigelow treats in tactful, even gingerly terms. If bleeding and purging and drugging are bad for sick people—if they may even be seen to hasten the death of the patient in many cases—why do physicians carry on with them? The answer at this preliminary stage has less to do with medicine than with human nature. In an earlier era, Galenic or humoral theory had been able to convince doctors that they were actually helping their patients. Today, when doubt has begun to set in, a doctor carries on because he does not want to admit his helplessness. Suppose, says Bigelow, that a friend falls ill: "we cannot stand by, as curious spectators. . . . We feel that we are called upon to attempt his rescue by vigorous means, so that at least the fault of omission shall not lie upon our charge." So the physician bleeds and purges, and if the patient gets even sicker, resorts to remedies he may only have heard of. Thus it normally occurs, says Bigelow, that "at the end of our attendance we may be left in uncertainty, whether the duration of sickness has been shortened, or lengthened, by our practice, and whether the patient is really indebted to us for good or evil."[72]

The other great question to be asked about self-limited disease is whether the physician who brings himself to believe in it must then, in a paralysis brought on by pure therapeutic skepticism, do no more than "fold his hands, and look passively on the progress of a disease, which he cannot interrupt"? Bigelow's answer is the same one given by most proponents of the *méthode expectante*: the physician is there to alleviate symptoms, and to take whatever measures might aid the body in its natural powers of recovery. Then, aware that he is addressing an American audience still reflexively loyal to that heroic medicine on which Benjamin Rush had set so memorable a stamp, Bigelow slyly points out that the *méthode expectante* has one incontestable advantage over rival approaches, which is that it permits the physician to save the patient from other doctors: "The opportunities of doing good may be as great in these diseases as in any others; for, in treating every disease, there is a right method, and a wrong. In the first place, we may save the patient from much harm, not only by forbearing ourselves to afflict him with unnecessary practice, but also by preventing the ill-judged activity of others."[73]

Oliver Wendell Holmes would spend much of his career as a medical writer expanding upon the principles set forth in his friend Dr. Bigelow's discourse on self-limited diseases. He would return to this particular point again and again, most often emphasizing something Bigelow leaves out: for patients who are sick but do not know what is happening to them, the physician's knowledge is in itself a powerful form of therapy. For the modern patient, this is the relief that comes when a biopsy or CAT scan turns out negative in what might have been a deadly disease. For the nineteenth-century patient, it was calling in a doctor who is able reliably to tell them what disease they have, and what to expect as it runs its course. "If every specific were to fail utterly," says Holmes in "Currents and Counter-Currents," if the cinchona trees all died out, and the arsenic mines were exhausted, . . . a body of enlightened men, organized as a distinct profession, would be required just as much as now, . . . to order all the conditions of the patient so as to favor the efforts of the system to right itself, and give those predictions of the course of disease which only experience can warrant, and which in so many cases relieve the exaggerated fears of sufferers and their friends."[74]

This is the moment in American medicine, in short, when the physician's authority was to be regrounded not in any sort of therapeutic measure at all, whether the massive bloodletting and purging of Rush's heroic practice, the botanical remedies of Thomsonian "popular" medicine, or the infinitesimal doses of the newly fashionable homeopathy, but simply and grandly in knowledge of what Holmes would once call "the natural progress of a malady, of its ordinary duration, of its various modes of terminating, of its liability to accidental complications, of the signs which mark its insignificance or its severity, of what is to be expected of it when left to itself, of how much or how little is to be anticipated from remedies."[75] Jacob Bigelow, a blunter soul, would make the point more tersely: "If a man has had the misfortune to get a shot or a stab in his body, he does not need a doctor who administers a specific dose or a sovereign plaster for holes in the body; he wants a man who can tell him whether the wound has passed inside or outside of his peritoneum, and whether it is requisite for him to make his will, or make arrangements for pursuing his journey."[76]

The address in which Bigelow makes this remark draws an analogy that may be taken as a summary statement of the principle, the great legacy to Boston medicine of Louis and the Paris clinical revolution, that only genuine medical knowledge may serve as a legitimate basis for medical authority and competence. Bigelow was on this occasion address-ing an audience of medical students. Most of them, he observes, carry a watch. When it stops, they never think of opening it up themselves to see what is wrong. They take it to an expert. The watchmaker may tell them that something moderately serious is wrong—a spring may be broken, a wheel need to be replaced—or that the problem is minor—the gears simply need oiling—or, if the watch has been seriously damaged in a fall or trodden underfoot, that it is beyond repair. All this comes from a competence that rests on knowledge and experience. But then, says Bigelow, suppose something else:

> Suppose there resides in the place a watch doctor who prescribes for symp-toms, and who, among other things, has a remedy for the symptom of stop-ping, and that this remedy consists in a certain kind of friction, shaking, or manipulation, an ointment applied to the outside, or an invisible particle of some nugatory substance inserted into the inside, and suppose that one or two watches in a hundred which had stopped by accident, should by accident resume their motions under such treatment, could anything but the most unmitigated folly draw the inference that such a person is enti-tled to become the accredited horologer to the community?[77]

The source of genuine medical authority is, in other words, as much moral as intellectual. For, as much as the continuous struggle against dis-ease to which every physician is called, medical competence also involves a ceaseless struggle against self-deception and dishonesty. Bigelow's views on self-deception we have already heard: a physician is a human being like any other, and when presented with the temptation to inter-vene in the name of medical expertise, is as liable to deceive himself as to deceive the patient. This is a note Holmes will strike again and again in his own medical writings, the way self-love and the fallacy of *post hoc ergo propter hoc*—"he got well after taking my medicine," as Holmes once tersely summarizes this error, "therefore in consequence of taking it"[78]—combine to create error: "Every sick person has done something or other by somebody's advice, or of his own accord, a little before get-ting better. There is an irresistible tendency to associate the thing done, and the improvement which followed it, as cause and effect. This is the great source of fallacy in medical practice. But the physician has some chance of correcting his hasty inference."[79]

Yet what if the physician, having been the source of the advice taken by the sick person just before he got well, takes credit for the cure? The point of Jacob Bigelow's analogy of the broken watch is precisely that a doctor is a genuine physician only if, knowing the true state of affairs, he makes no attempt to deceive the patient. Bigelow puts the choice in stark terms to the audience of young medical students he is addressing. Those of his listeners who go forth with their degrees and pursue medicine as "a liberal and honorable science, to be followed for the good it may do to mankind," are real physicians. They may be depended upon to increase their knowledge of medicine as time goes on, through study and experience, and to practice their calling "with conscience and fidelity." The others, who prescribe meaningless or dangerous remedies, or who permit patients to believe that it was the doctor, rather than nature, who brought about their healing, are parasites and charlatans. Such a one, says Bigelow, practices medicine "as a dishonest trade, to be pursued for the purpose of profiting himself by the deception of his fellow-men." His only increase in knowledge will be in "the low arts which entrap the credulous and unwary."[80]

Jacob Bigelow was an unmetaphysical soul, someone who thought of himself as a dealer in plain truths and wholesome common sense. Yet even he is not always able to avoid a metaphysical language in stating his case. "The longer and the more philosophically we contemplate this subject," he says in his address on self-limited diseases, "the more obvious it will appear, that the physician is but the minister and servant of nature; that . . . we can do little more than follow in the train of disease, and endeavor to aid nature in her salutary intentions."[81] Here we have the rediscovery in Boston, under the influence of Paris medicine, of the ancient principle of the *vis medicatrix naturae*, the healing power of nature, and by extension, a principle that creates and sustains life in a universe otherwise ruled by death and decay. One effect of Paris study on Mason Warren, says Howard Payson Arnold, was the "gradual diminution in the quantity of medicine he prescribed, and his constantly increasing faith in the *vis medicatrix naturae*."[82] We encounter the same principle in similar terms in William Paley's immensely influential *Natural Theology*, a work never far from Holmes's mind when he is writing about either of his two great subjects, medicine and religion:

> The other property of our nature, to which we are still more beholden, is its constant endeavour to restore itself, when disordered, to its regular course. The fluids of the body appear to possess a power of separating and expelling any noxious substance which may have mixed with them. This they do in eruptive fevers, by a kind of despumation, as Sydenham calls it. . . . The solids, on their part, when their action is obstructed, not only resume that action, as soon as the obstruction is removed, but they struggle with the impediment. They take an action as near to the true one, as the difficulty and the organization, with which they have to contend, will allow of.[83]

Oliver Wendell Holmes in Paris

To observe the gradual emergence of the *vis medicatrix naturae* as the central principle of Boston medicine is to glimpse an answer to that question Sir William Osler did not think to address a hundred years ago: why did P. C. A. Louis—and, in the background, the teachings of La Charité from Bayle and Laennec through Chomel, Andral, and Louis himself—exert so strong an influence on American students? The answer, it will now appear, lies in a crucial distinction. For Louis's impact on such American students as the Philadelphian William Gerhard simply involved his role as representative of the anatomico-pathological medicine that had begun with Bichat. Gerhard would return to Philadelphia to pursue recognizably "Parisian" researches that would make him famous as the first pathologist to distinguish reliably between typhoid and typhus fever, two utterly different diseases with different courses and different prognoses, but easily confused with each other during the onset stage.[84] Yet Louis's influence on Boston students would be, as we have seen, primarily in the direction of the *méthode expectante* and a trust, confirmed by rigorous empirical analysis, in the *vis medicatrix naturae*. So, to rephrase the question, why did the teachings of Louis have such an impact on this singularly gifted group of students from, specifically, Boston?

The answer, it is reasonable to suppose, had a great deal to do with Boston itself, and in particular with a civic culture that provided a locus of resistance to the irresistible spread of a raw economic individualism elsewhere coming to dominance in Jacksonian America. The image of Boston that emerges in the extraordinary two-volume *Life of John Collins Warren* written by his son Edward, for instance—a neglected classic both of early American medical literature and of social and intellectual history—will immediately suggest to any serious student of Paris medicine why young men like James Jackson, Jr., Henry Bowditch, Oliver Wendell Holmes, and Warren's own son Mason so insistently felt the gravitational pull of Louis's clinical teaching at La Pitié, dedicated to the pursuit of truth for its own sake, and to medicine as the very symbol of, in Jacob Bigelow's phrase, a liberal and honorable science. Boston was in this sense a special case of the more general difference Tocqueville had remarked between the Eastern states, where institutions obeyed a rule of "wisdom and durability," while "in the Western states, on the contrary, society seems to be ruled by chance."[85] In the Boston of the 1830s, Henry Adams would similarly observe, "the logical social results of republican institutions had not yet worked themselves out. Lingering tradition and close-woven associations seemed solid and sure to continue."[86]

The same civic temper does a great deal to explain why this group of Boston medical students would become leaders in the movement towards trust in the *vis medicatrix naturae*. For the overwhelming tension in Paris medicine when they studied there had been between speculative systems rooted in revolutionary ideology and a more traditional wisdom insisting that nature, however slow to reveal her secrets, was the only sound basis of medical practice. This is the context in which, for instance, Stephen Jacyna views the combat between Broussais and the school of La Charité as mirroring in medical terms the ideological conflict between the Jacobin radicals in the French Revolution and the Burke of *Reflections on the Revolution in France*, so witheringly contemptuous of schemes for remaking human society in the name of this or that purely abstract doctrine. There is, as Jacyna points out, something inescapably Burkean in François Chomel's insistence that, revolutionary medical systems notwithstanding, wisdom comes only from a deep recognition that nature works in slow and intricate ways:

> In the midst of the revolutions that physiological theories have undergone and the alterations they have entailed in the practice of the majority of physicians, the symptoms and the progress of the disease have not changed. The observations of physicians who have studied faithfully the process of nature have not aged. . . . Alien to all species of system, we have never entertained any opinion, at any time, either upon the special seat, or the intimate nature of the disease that occupies us. We have confined ourselves to following attentively the phenomena and the progress, and to examining the effect of the means that we have seen employed, or that we have ourselves put into use. If this disposition does not protect against all error, it is at least fitted to distance us from that form of bias which makes it improper to observe.[87]

In speaking of revolutions in clinical practice Chomel was, of course, talking about Broussais. Taken as an epitome of the teachings of *l'école de La Charité*, especially as they would take on greater weight from Louis's researches on bloodletting, Chomel's remarks do much to explain why Boston physicians were so ready to turn against the therapeutic regimen instituted by Benjamin Rush, whom Ackerknecht correctly characterized as an American version of Broussais.[88] It serves as well to explain Holmes's special alertness to the relation between Rush's democratic ideology and the theories Rush invented to justify his own heroic practice. Jacksonian democracy was the culmination of a movement whose origins lay in Thomas Jefferson's unrepentant sympathy for Jacobin radicalism.[89] In a Jacksonian America in which every patient has the right to expect his physician's aggressive intervention against the malignant forces of "nature," was it, indeed, any wonder to see the stars and stripes waving over doses of ninety grains of sulphate of quinine, and the American eagle screaming with delight to see three drachms of calomel given at a single mouthful? To oppose such doctrines, on the other hand, was precisely to view the physician as, in Bigelow's phrase, the minister and servant of nature.

As Tocqueville would clearly see, there is always in such cases an essential relation between political democracy and, in a society driven by the marketplace, a tendency to be taken in by charlatanism. A feature of American democracy is that every citizen feels the tremendous weight of a pressure to conform to public opinion—"it does not persuade others to its beliefs," observed Tocqueville, "but it imposes them and makes them permeate the thinking of everyone by a sort of enormous pressure of the mind of all upon the individual intelligence"[90]— without ever thinking to ask whether that opinion is well or ill founded. It takes a long time and much discrimination, Tocqueville remarks, to arrive at a true estimate of the character even of a single individual. Under the conditions of American democracy, "the people have neither the time nor the means for an investigation of this kind. Their conclusions are hastily formed from a superficial inspection of the more prominent features of a question. Hence it often happens that mountebanks of all sorts are able to please the people, while their truest friends frequently fail to win their confidence."[91]

Holmes would devote a great deal of his career as a medical writer to combating medical charlatanism, in a Jacksonian America where Tocqueville's mountebank might appear in the guise of a Thomsonian "people's doctor," a homeopathist with a foreign or American diploma, or a regularly-educated physician who against all evidence had refused to give up the bleeding, purging, drugging regimen instituted by Rush in the 1790s. In a world where the pressures of the marketplace gave doctors an incentive to treat disease, as one nineteenth-century physician put it, "in great measure according to the desire of their patients,"[92] the only recourse of the *médecine expectant* lay in a reasoned defense of its basis in genuine medical knowledge. Even the known terrors of massive bloodletting were not enough to discourage patients taught to associate venesection with "real" medical intervention. A patient entering the hospital in 1844, reports John Harley Warner, told his attendants that he had "been accustomed to be bled very year, about this time"; the attending physician ordered that 18 ounces of blood be removed. Similarly, the records of an Irish farmer entering Massachusetts General Hospital at about the same time record that he was "very anxious to be bled."[93]

The purest expression of the Jacksonian medical marketplace was the market in patent medicines. Such medicines were not, of course, in any sense peculiarly American. Itinerant mountebanks had wandered the roads of medieval and early modern Europe—they were, reported Frances Trollope, still highly visible in Paris in the early nineteenth century[94]—and patent medicine advertisements appear in the earliest

newspapers published in eighteenth-century London. Yet their prolif-
eration in Jacksonian America was a matter of common remark. Holmes, for instance, tells the story of a fellow physician who saw a patient
who had come to him with a severe soreness in his mouth: "On inquiry
he found that the man had picked up a box of unknown pills, in Howard Street, and had proceeded to take them, on general principles, pills
being good for people." As it happens, the pills contained mercury, with
what effects we have seen. Yet, as Holmes is aware, the man was merely
the creature of a medical marketplace in which the *vox populi* is now
understood in terms mainly of consumer preference: "Somebody buys
all the quack medicines that build palaces for the mushroom, say rather,
the toadstool millionaires. Who is it? These people have a constituency
of millions."[95]

Lectures like Holmes's *Homeopathy and Its Kindred Delusions* would
thus participate in a movement that would make Boston and its immediate environs a center of resistance not simply to the dominance of
market forces in nineteenth-century America, but to an ideology that
ceaselessly proclaimed these forces as the purest expression of American
democracy. In works like Thoreau's *Walden* and Emerson's lectures—
"When I . . . speak of the democratic element," declared Emerson, "I do
not mean that ill thing, vain and loud, which writes lying newspapers,
spouts at caucuses, and sells its lies for gold; . . . There is nothing of
the true democratic element in what is called Democracy; it must fall,
being wholly commercial."[96]— this critique would be incorporated into
literary Transcendentalism. In the politically engaged atmosphere of the
Abolitionist period, it would be heard as well from the pulpit. "Wealth is
the great object of American desire," remarked Theodore Parker. "Cov-
etousness is the American passion. This is so—nationally in the political
affairs of the country; ecclesiastically, socially, domestically, individually."
In America, Parker said, money "is counted as the end of life, not as the
material basis to the higher forms thereof."[97]

Yet outside of Boston, especially in the South of Jefferson and Madison and the backwoods strongholds of Jacksonian democracy, such sentiments would be heard as anti-democratic condescension, the attempt
of a self-appointed "aristocracy" to assert the superiority of its values over
that of a population simply doing its best to fulfil its material ambitions.
"Men who live in democratic communities," Tocqueville had observed,
"not only seldom indulge in meditation, but they naturally entertain very
little esteem for it."[98] "There is no class in America," he remarked elsewhere, "in which the taste for intellectual pleasures is transmitted with
hereditary fortune and leisure and by which the labors of the intellect
are held in honor."[99] When the voice of such a class began to be heard
in Boston in the 1830s, it would inevitably be heard not as an expres-

sion of intellectual values but as a mere attempt to assert social superiority. "Now how shall it be written?" asks the narrator of Mrs. Harrison Gray Otis, Jr.'s novel *The Barclays of Boston.* "That the Bartons were not of the same rank as the Barclays,—no such word as rank in democratic America. Not of the same class,—that will never do. . . . The fact is, and the truth must be told, it is very hard, indeed, to describe certain things in America."[100]

Nonetheless, the Boston to which Holmes returned in 1834 well knew that its resistance to the economic individualism of Jacksonian democracy—what Emerson meant when, looking at the America around him, he cried out that man had become "a money chest": "He is the servant of his belly. This is the casual bankruptcy, this is the cruel oppression"[101]— was not in any true sense based on feelings of social superiority. Indeed, its greatest pride was precisely in an intellectual culture in which talent or intelligence, as George Ticknor had once approvingly said about Edinburgh, "breaks down all the artificial distinctions of society."[102] Still, this was a truth that could be uttered only by Bostonians to other Bostonians, as in Howard Payson Arnold's privately-printed memoir of Mason Warren: "Taken as a whole its citizens held a rank much above the average for morality and intelligence, for thrift, energy, and public spirit. . . . As the people were for the most part well educated and read much, there was no subject of popular concern on which they failed to have views of their own or thought themselves incompetent to offer an opinion. As they had long been broadly patriotic, they easily identified themselves with the well-being of the whole nation."[103]

So it was that Oliver Wendell Holmes, who would come to be more strongly identified with Boston than any other writer, would discover in the apparently removed area of medical controversy the possibility of a literary idiom in which staunch resistance to a Jacksonian money or market society might be proclaimed without giving offense to the larger American public. The rallying cry in the name of which he would be permitted to denounce such popular movements as homeopathy, all the while subjecting the errors of an ignorant populace to withering logical scrutiny, would be the *vis medicatrix naturae*, a power more ancient than any city or civilization. "We who are on the side of 'Nature' please ourselves," he could confidently declare in "Currents and Counter-Currents in Medical Science," "that we are in the great current in which the true intelligence of the time is moving. We believe that some who oppose, or fear, or denounce our movement are themselves caught in various eddies that set back against the truth. . . . If there is any State or city which might claim to be the American headquarters of the nature-trusting heresy, provided it be one, that State is Massachusetts, and that city is its capital."[104]

As we shall see, the literary career launched with Holmes's small treatise on the contagiousness of puerperal fever would rise, first through medical discourses like "Currents and Counter-Currents in Medical Science," then through more consciously popular works like *Homeopathy and its Kindred Delusions*, to the apogee signaled by the appearance of *The Autocrat of the Breakfast Table* in the *Atlantic Monthly* in 1857. Yet through every stage of this career, sustained by a literary voice whose endlessly witty ebullience is matched nowhere else in American writing, the tutelary spirit hovering over Holmes's writing table would the modest Paris physician whose rounds he had once followed in the wards of La Pitié. "You ought to know," he wrote in a private letter to Emerson, who had made the grievous mistake of mentioning Louis in public as an example of French theatricality, "that Louis never *succeeded* in France until Americans gave him a name. . . . He assimilated to himself many of the best and most laborious students . . . but there was nothing to keep them around him except his truthfulness, diligence, and *modesty in the presence of nature.*" The "master key to all the success he ever had," Holmes concludes, ". . . was honesty."[105] During the writing of the Breakfast Table trilogy, it would always be Louis who symbolized for Holmes what one character in *The Poet of the Breakfast Table* would call the absolute and utter *humility* of science—the one great principle that would sustain Holmes in his unending battle against pride and presumption in theology and politics as well as medicine.

CHAPTER FOUR

The Spirit of Paris

*I*n the years immediately after Holmes's return from Paris, Jacob Big-elow would remain the primary spokesman for therapeutic skepti-cism, his "On Self-Limited Diseases" the bible of the *médecine expectante* as it would come to be associated primarily with Boston and, within the Bos-ton medical community, with Harvard Medical School and the Tremont Street Medical School at which both Holmes and Bigelow gave private instruction. But gradually, as Holmes's fame as an author grew, he would take over this role from his senior colleague. The best-known apothegm ever delivered against the drugging system would be a casual witticism delivered by Holmes in "Currents and Counter-Currents in Medical Sci-ence," delivered before the Massachusetts Medical Society in May, 1860: "Throw out opium, which the Creator himself seems to prescribe. . . ; throw out a few specifics which our art did not discover, and is hardly needed to apply; throw out wine, which is a food, and the vapors which produce the miracle of anæsthesis, and I firmly believe that if the whole materia medica, *as now used*, could be sunk to the bottom of the sea, it would be all the better for mankind,—and all the worse for the fishes."[1]

The epigrammatic turn of the last sentence made it instantly famous. The final phrase, Holmes would recall thirty years later, "was misquoted, quoted without its qualifying conditions, and frightened some of my worthy professional brethren as much as if I had told them to throw all physic to the dogs."[2] Some of Holmes's colleagues in the Massachu-setts Medical Society met the day after the address was delivered to vote through a public statement dissociating themselves from the sentiment it expressed.[3] Yet by and large the Boston medical community had come to agree with the *méthode expectante* as the only rational mode of treat-ment in an epoch when discoveries were constantly being made at the level of basic science—in "Border Lines of Knowledge in Medical Sci-ence," for instance, delivered to the medical class at Harvard a year later, Holmes would give a superb account of the revolution in histology brought about by the new compound microscope[4]—but therapeutic measures had remained unaltered virtually since the days of Galen. This is the context in which, in his medical writings over the next decades, Holmes's emphasis would gradually shift to emphasize the *vis medicatrix naturae* as the mysterious power of healing that was revealed in all its majesty when the expectant method was employed in therapy.

The *vis medicatrix* would become for Holmes a vital metaphysical principle, the ground he would occupy against both the grim New England theology of his boyhood and the new climate of Victorian religious anxiety created by science and philosophical materialism. As we have seen, materialist philosophy had been a major impetus for the new Paris clinical medicine. It was popularly associated among medical students with outspoken materialists like Broussais, but was also an important element of scientific belief for less flamboyant souls like Corvisart. Indeed, Corvisart at about the same time as he was introducing percussion as a diagnostic method at La Charité was, as W. R. Albury notes, an uncompromising spokesman for nature as a blind and destructive force, the very opposite of anything that could be seen as a *vis medicatrix*. Some doctors, observed Corvisart, maintain that nature tries to establish an equilibrium where it does not exist, but "impartial observation gives the lie to this exaggerated solicitude of nature, this restorative and corrective spirit of the vital principle." The "errors of nature," he claimed, "are perhaps both more frequent and more fatal" than her attempts to heal.[5]

In the eighteenth century, the same intellectual climate that had produced the religious skepticism of Voltaire and the atheism of Helvetius and Holbach produced a response to that skepticism in what is usually called physico-theology, the inspiration for which was found in Newton's *Principia*. For Newton, in proving that the entire material universe was governed by a simple set of physical laws—that the apple in one's hand and the most distant galaxies equally obey the law of gravitation, for instance—and that these laws could be elegantly expressed in a few mathematical formulas, had inspired that Deism that in the salons of the French Enlightenment would come to seem the most rational alternative to an outmoded Christianity, with its improbable tales of miracle-working and casting-out of devils and resurrection from the dead. The most radical version of the Unitarianism that would eventually triumph in Boston was essentially Deism of this sort, and Holmes, as a prominent spokesman for its liberal theology, has sometimes mistakenly been seen as an eighteenth-century Deist who had simply expanded his physico-theology to accommodate the new teachings of Lyell in geology or Darwin in evolutionary biology.

At the heart of physico-theology, in turn, was the argument from design: the proposition that the laws of nature are at once so complex and so uniform that it is wholly improbable to attribute them to blind chance. The most famous version of this argument was that given by William Paley in *Natural Theology* (1802). A man walking across a heath comes upon a watch lying on the ground. The stone lying next to it may plausibly be understood as the product of blind material forces working without aim or purpose. But the watch, once one has seen that it tells time, and that the chances against this particular arrangement of wheels and springs and gears having come together for that purpose by pure random chance are vanishingly small, argues the existence of a watch-maker: the "clockmaker God" who would figure so largely in later histories of Deism. Yet Paley, though he is best known for this mechanical analogy, in reality drew his main inspiration as a theologian from biology and comparative anatomy. *Natural Theology*, Sir William Osler would say, speaking of Elisha Bartlett's 1839 edition of Paley's work, "was really a delightful commentary on anatomy and physiology" and thus for students of his own generation "a happy change from artificial theology."[6]

Paley's shift of the argument from design to the living world was momentous in its implications for younger physicians like Holmes and Elisha Bartlett. For what the eighteenth-century Deists had not seen, in their initial entrancement with the newly-revealed Newtonian cosmology, was that their physico-theology preserved the essential notion of a dead material universe. An infinite space populated by stars and galaxies in endless motion was, no matter how mathematically elegant and intricate, a universe oblivious to human existence. Paley's *Natural Theology* does, it is true, make a point of honoring the premises of the older Deism, whose principle of cosmic intelligibility it needs for its own purposes. "The same order of things attends us wherever we go," he observes. "The elements act upon one another, electricity operates, the tides rise and fall, the magnet needle elects its position in one region of the earth as well as in another. . . . one sun illuminates; one moon exerts its specific attraction upon all parts."[7] Gravitation, he similarly remarks elsewhere, "though everywhere around us, near us, and within us; though diffused throughout all space, and penetrating the texture of all bodies with which we are acquainted . . . is no object of sense to us."[8]

Nonetheless, Paley is aware that, given future discoveries in physics, materialists might declare the dead universe to be wholly intelligible on grounds implying neither intelligence nor design on the part of a Creator. This is the spirit in which, for instance, he denounces Buffon's hypothesis of "organic particles"—the eighteenth-century version of the electric spark that creates life from a primal soup—as nothing more than the ancient atomism of Democritus in modern disguise. For on what principle could atoms and molecules in a whirl of blind motion

produce living beings? Buffon had hypothesized that the earth was created and set in motion when a comet broke off part of the sun. But then,
as Paley points out, he needs another sort of hypothesis to create plants
and animals. "In order to solve this difficulty, we are to suppose the universe replenished with particles endowed with life, but without organiza-
tion or sense of their own, and endowed also with a tendency to marshall
themselves into organized forms. The concourse of these particles, by
virtue of this tendency, but without intelligence, will, or direction . . . has
produced the living forms which we now see."[9]

The major weakness of Paley's argument, as Holmes among others
would perceive, is that it could be demolished by any hypothesis that
could explain the same facts on purely physical principles, without
recourse to intelligent design. So, for instance, given the right set of circumstances, it might be shown that organic molecules are able be formed
from inorganic compounds, along with a means of replication. This, and
not its more obvious conflict with the story of creation as recounted in
Genesis, is what made Darwinism so powerful a threat to nineteenth-
century religious belief. The principle of natural selection can explain,
as elegantly as Paley's notion of intelligent design, the hare's backbone
and the human eye, and for every example of miraculous contrivance
or complexity in *Natural Theology* there is a Darwinian counter-example
that needs only the principle of nature as, in the phrase of one modern
evolutionist, a blind watchmaker. This is why Holmes, though sympathetic to the sort of point Paley was trying to make, seldom gives him
more than a passing mention in his medical writings. For long before
Darwin published *The Origin of Species*, Holmes had seen that the argument from design was, on its own terms, vulnerable to purely scientific
invalidation.

The alternative that would gain Holmes's allegiance, that would leave
him entranced with the discoveries of geology and paleontology, and
that would permit him to absorb new systems like Darwinism painlessly
into an already-developed structure of belief, was the notion of scientific
theories as a new form of revelation, not simply about the physical universe but about the nature of human consciousness. For the weak point
of purely physical explanation appeared to be that, even as it accounted
for the laws by which planets circle the sun, or species ascend the scale
from trilobites to pterodactyls to mastodons, it gave no obvious account
of the consciousness able to postulate such laws, or of the collective consciousness, sustained by language and social institutions, in whose mental universe theories like Darwin's played so significant a role. Nor did it
seem possible for the human consciousness that devised such theories to
discover a point outside itself—in, precisely, that blind whirl of matter in
which thought or language or logic do not exist—to account for its own

existence. On this ground, of a universe becoming more and more intelligible to a consciousness that remains unexplained by its own theories of atomic bonding or natural selection, Holmes would situate his own metaphysics.

For medical students in Paris, the notion of science as a new mode of divine revelation was most commonly associated with Cuvier's studies in comparative anatomy, which seemed so insistently to suggest a proto-Darwinian view of evolutionary relationships, and in particular with the anatomical museum at the Jardin des Plantes. To people living in previous ages, exclaimed Augustus Gardner, "a sudden introduction to such a universe, though but in miniature as the Garden of Plants presents, would have disclosed an absolutely new creation." Even in the nineteenth century, such a microcosm cannot be viewed "without experiencing, as it were, a new revelation of the Creator, in the unexpected lights, that burst upon the spectator, of the relations and design of his omnipotent productions. What was before imagined to be a chaos of chance is proved to be the symmetry of a fixed purpose."[10] The language is that of Paley's *Natural Theology*—"Under this stupendous Being we live," Paley had similarly exclaimed: "in every portion of nature, which we can descry, we find attention bestowed upon even the minutest parts"[11]—but the notion of science as a new revelation is very close to Holmes.

The difference is that Holmes would always emphasize science as a mode of revelatory speech or language intelligible to human consciousness—the stubborn fact that sticks and stones are not aware, so to speak, of the laws by which they fall to the ground—and therefore as an evident form of participation in a higher realm of intelligence. "To fear science or knowledge, lest it disturb our old beliefs," Holmes would argue, "is to fear the influx of the Divine wisdom into the souls of our fellow-man, for what is science but the piece-meal *revelation*— uncovering—of the plan of creation, by the agency of those chosen prophets of nature whom God has illuminated from the central light of truth for that single purpose?"[12] In the same spirit, he will speak of fossil discoveries as "those new tables of the law, placed in the hands of the geologist by the same living God who spoke from Sinai to the Israelites of old,"[13] and argue in a late essay that "theology, the science of Him whom by searching no man can find out, is fast being replaced by what we may not improperly call theonomy, or the science of the laws according to which the Creator acts."[14]

The moments in his medical essays at which Holmes seems most like an eighteenth-century Deist are those in which he emphasizes the sublimity of an infinite universe governed by rational laws. This is the spirit in which, for instance, he gives as an echo of his own thoughts a passage from Burdach's *Physiologie*: "There is for me but one miracle, that of infinite existence, and but one mystery, the manner in which the finite proceeds from the infinite. So soon as we recognize this incomprehensible act as the general and primordial miracle, of which our reason perceives the necessity, but the manner of which our intelligence cannot grasp, . . . there is for us no other impenetrable miracle or mystery."[15] The moments at which he sounds least like a conventional Deist, on the other hand, are those in which he contemplates the healing powers of nature, as when a treatise on the management of compound fractures of the leg provides the occasion for a positively lyrical outburst, as providing incontestable evidence of "the supreme wisdom, forethought, and adaptive dexterity of that divine Architect, as shown in repairing the shattered columns which support the living temple of the body."[16]

The latter voice belongs to the essential Holmes, the physician who has again and again seen the *vis medicatrix naturae* working in opposition to disease, decay, and death, and for whom it has thus come to represent not simply a scientific but a moral fact about the order of the universe. This gives us the context in which *The Autocrat of the Breakfast Table* and the later Breakfast Table volumes demand to be read, not as religious works, but, as with Carlyle's *Sartor Resartus* or Tennyson's *In Memoriam*, as works in which an older theological vocabulary remains indispensable to any inquiry into the modern condition. No better guide to the contemporary response to Holmes's writing can be found, to my mind, than Paley's observations on this subject: "The train of spontaneous thought, and the choice of that train, may be directed to different ends, . . . but *in a moral view*, I shall not, I believe, be contradicted when I say, that, if one train of thinking be more desirable than another, it is that which regards the phenomena of nature with a constant reference to a supreme intelligent Author. To have made this the ruling, the habitual sentiment of our minds, is to have laid the foundation of everything which is religious."[17]

The foundations of Holmes's religious or metaphysical speculation in the Breakfast Table trilogy and elsewhere lie in the conception of a Creator whose moral relation to humankind is disclosed in the power that opposes birth, growth, and healing to the destructive forces of death, decay, and disintegration. Of what is evil in human life—hunger, pain, destruction—a great deal is produced by human beings themselves, as in the case of war and rapine, and much else—natural calamities, the suffering of infants—it is beyond the power of human intelligence to grasp. The important point is that the Creator encountered by the doctor in his daily rounds, and especially by the physician wise enough to have adopted the *médecine expectante*, is, as Holmes puts it, "the Being whom Ambroise Paré meant when he spoke those memorable words, which you may read over the professor's chair in the French School of Medicine,—"*Je le pensay, et Dieu le guarit*,"— "I dressed the wound, and God healed it." The God of whom Paré was speaking, as Holmes wryly remarks, is a somewhat "different being from the God that scholastic theologians have projected from their consciousness."[18]

The story of Ambroise Paré is virtually a parable of the *vis medicatrix naturae* as it had providentially revealed itself to the great sixteenth-century French surgeon. For Paré, like Velpeau in Holmes's day a peasant boy from the provinces who had risen by virtue of pure talent and industry, was like most surgeons of that violent time called upon to practice on the battlefield. The standard treatment for wounds called for pouring on boiling oil of elder, a torture to men already in agonizing pain. On one occasion, Paré's supply of oil ran out. He treated the wounds of his soldiers with a mild ointment of his own making. Holmes tells the story: "He could not sleep that night for fear his patients who had not been scalded with the boiling oil would be poisoned by the gunpowder conveyed into their wounds by the balls. To his surprise, he found them much better than the others the next morning, and resolved never again to burn his patients with hot oil for gunshot wounds."[19] "*Je le pensay, et Dieu le guarit,*"—this is the context in which Holmes will be able seriously to claim that medical science in his own time "is destined . . . to react to much greater advantage on the theology of the future than theology has acted on medicine in the past."[20]

Yet medical science, as it entered theology by way of Holmes's pen, would not do so without controversy. For religious views based on the *vis medicatrix naturae*, positing a benign or benevolent order in the universe, would put Holmes on a violent collision course not only with the New England theology of his childhood, but with a Calvinist orthodoxy that retained a powerful intellectual influence through his early years as a physician and author. The angry God of Jonathan Edwards was still the presiding deity of the New England to which Holmes returned from his studies in Paris, and the battle against the doctrines of innate depravity and predestination would not be won without dust and heat. As we shall see, Holmes speaking as a physician was able to posit the existence of a benign universe and a benevolent Creator in a way that gave his Breakfast Table books a special and important status in the literature of Victorian religious anxiety. It was, on the other hand, the ferocity with which he would always insist on treating New England theology as a spiritual disease that for many contemporary readers lent his writings, underneath their surface of wit and pleasantry and imperturbable geniality, a dangerous edge.

No better introduction be found to what I shall be calling Holmes's *religio medici* than his treatment of New England Puritanism in "The Medical Profession in Massachusetts," a lecture delivered at the Lowell Institute in 1869. For there the Calvinism of the Puritan fathers is treated in its historical setting as a curiosity of a naive and credulous age, not essentially different from the remedies they used to cure plague, smallpox, fevers, falling-sickness, or the king's evil. Thus, for instance, Governor Winthrop no doubt believed in the innate depravity of man and the guilt of children born under Adam's curse, but so did he believe in a marvellous powder—good "against the plague, small-pox; purples, all sorts of feavers; Poyson; either by Way of Prevention or after Infection"[21]—made by filling an earthen pot with live toads, baking the pot over a fire, then pounding the dessicated toads until they were reduced first into a brown, and then into a black powder. Other conditions were treated with rhubarb or jalap, or, Holmes reports, having examined the medical records of the early colonies, occasionally "an electuary of *millipedes*—sowbugs, if we must give them their honest English name."[22]

By the time Holmes's account of New England medicine gets to Cotton Mather in the early eighteenth century, however, the doctrines of innate depravity and predestination no longer have the excuse of belonging to a barbarous or credulous epoch. For Mather was the creature of a rational age, someone living after Locke and Newton, aware enough of the medical science of his time to have introduced inoculation against smallpox to New England. Yet he was also, by choice, a hanger of witches and a tireless promulgator of the same Calvinist doctrines that his forebears had brought with them to the New World along with their recipes for toad powder. Having been a polymath and an incurable busybody, he had also written medical texts for the use of his flock. The governing principle is theological: disease is the effect of sin. "So saying," as Holmes reports, "he encourages the young mother whose babe is wasting away on her breast with these reflections:—"

> "Think of the grievous Effects of *Sin!* This wretched *Infant* has not yet arrived unto years of sense enough, to *sin after the similitude of the transgression committed by Adam.* Nevertheless the *Transgression of Adam,* who had all mankind *Fœderally,* yea, Naturally, in him, has involved this Infant in the guilt of it. And the *poison of the old serpent,* which infected *Adam* when he fell into his *Transgression,* by hearkening to the Tempter, has corrupted all mankind, and is a seed unto such diseases as this *Infant* is now laboring under. *Lord,* what are we, and what are our children, but a Generation of Vipers?"[23]

Holmes's answer was that disease was a physical event. Nor does Mather's Calvinism explain why the vast majority of illnesses to which human beings are subject get better by themselves. The child's chicken pox or measles pass by, bestowing immunity as they go. The shivers and fever of an adult in the grip of an influenza end in a few days. The broken leg mends itself, the wound heals. To Holmes, it would always be the

Oliver Wendell Holmes in Paris

regenerative power that works toward healing that served to expose the angry God of New England theology as a monstrous projection of human presumption and theological error. His own Paris medical studies, and the growing importance of the *vis medicatrix naturae* to the Boston students who had walked the wards of La Pitié with P. C. A. Louis, had made it impossible to believe that the Creator of the universe had, as Holmes says in one of his essays, doomed infants like those described by Cotton Mather to a place of torment "where no organ finds itself in its natural medium, where no wound heals kindly," and "where the omnipotent is unfelt save in malignant agencies." The physician's God, says Holmes, is one who "never leaves himself without witness, who repenteth him of the evil, who never allows a disease or an injury . . . to take its course without establishing an effort . . . always, to restore the broken body or the shattered mind."[24]

The story of Holmes's emergence as a major nineteenth-century American author begins in the medical writings he began to compose shortly after his return from Paris. The most important of these originated in a paper delivered to a small group of fellow Boston physicians. On February 13, 1843, Holmes addressed the Society for Medical Improvement on the subject of puerperal fever, a dreaded infection that attacked women who had just given birth. In large cities like London, Paris, and Vienna, the disease was associated with the lying-in hospitals established to accommodate an expanding urban population. Within the walls of such hospitals was generated a miasma, Holmes grimly reminded his listeners, as "deadly in some institutions as the plague; which has killed women in a private hospital of London so fast that they were buried two in one coffin to conceal its horrors; which enabled Tonnellé to record two hundred and twenty-two autopsies at the Maternité of Paris," and "which has led Dr. Lee to express his deliberate conviction that the loss of life occasioned by these institutions completely defeats the objects of their founders."[25] Holmes's object in his talk to the Society was to convince physicians in his own city, most of whom still delivered babies at home, that even in these supposedly safer circumstances women were very often dying because the doctor himself was carrying the disease to the bedside.

Nearly half a century later, when Pasteur's discoveries had led to the germ theory of disease, Holmes would remark to Sir William Osler that he was pleased to have taken his ground on the existing evidence "before the little army of microbes was marched up" to support his position.[26] At the time his talk was delivered, the cause of the illness was utterly mysterious. Its effects, however, were all too well known. "It commonly begins," reported *The London Practice of Physic* in 1779, "with a rigor or chilliness, on the first, second, or third day after delivery; followed by a violent pain, and soreness, over the whole hypogastric region. There is much thirst; pain in the head, chiefly in the forehead, and parts about the eyebrows; a flushing in the face; anxiety, a hot dry skin; quick and weak pulse . . . a shortness in breathing . . . When the disease proves fatal, a diarrhœa generally supervenes."[27] Very often, the newborn child came down with the illness as well, usually with fatal results. The question, especially for physicians with a large obstetric practice, as well for as those teaching obstetrics to medical students, was why some women were vulnerable to the disease while others remained untouched.

The means by which the illness was being transmitted to parturient women by their doctors would be isolated in Vienna by Ignaz Philipp Semmelweis in Vienna only four years after Holmes delivered his talk in Boston. As Semmelweis would do, Holmes postulated a connection between childbed fever and anatomical dissection. Physicians who nicked themselves with a scalpel when performing autopsies on puerperal women, for instance, were known to have gotten ill with a disease exactly like puerperal fever. If they died, the symptoms and stages of the illness were identical. In other cases, physicians who had suffered a succession of serious or fatal puerperal cases in their own practice had turned out to have visited households where erysipelas was present. In the same way, Holmes's research in the medical literature turned up evidence very like that from which Semmelweis would draw his conclusions several years later. Thus, for instance, he cites Rigby's *System of Midwifery*: "That the discharges from a patient under puerperal fever are in the highest degree contagious we have abundant evidence in the history of lying-in hospitals. The puerperal abscesses are also contagious, and may be communicated to healthy lying-in women by washing with the same sponge; this fact has been repeatedly proved in the Vienna Hospital."[28]

Holmes's great problem was that, in a city where most women were delivered at home, the argument that puerperal fever was being carried by doctors or midwives from childbed to childbed had to be purely circumstantial, and moreover to deal with chance variations that seemed to defy a logic of numerical correlation. Throughout his tireless campaign to establish the truth of puerperal contagiousness, Holmes would be plagued by what he came to call "negative facts." A physician whose practice had produced a number of puerperal fatalities within a limited period of time, for instance, would also have delivered a number of women who did *not* come down with the illness. How did a theory of contagion, especially one claiming that the physician going from bedside to bedside carried the illness with him, propose to explain why a doctor visiting patients in identical circumstances transmitted the disease to some of them and not to others? Was it not more reasonable to assume, in such cases, that some other factor common to the afflicted women, but having nothing to do with the physician, was responsible for their illness?

Holmes was supremely logical even in the most casual of his writings. "The Contagiousness of Puerperal Fever" would provide his own education in dealing with opponents inept at logical reasoning. ("I had a savage pleasure," he would later tell Osler, speaking of the two most prominent opponents of his argument, "in handling those two professors—learned men both of them, skilful experts, but babies, as it seemed to me, in their capacity of reasoning and arguing.")[29] His first move in the talk originally delivered to his medical colleagues in Boston had been to set aside as irrelevant all questions about *what* is responsible for carrying the illness from patient to patient: "I shall not enter into any dispute about the particular *mode* of infection, whether it be by the atmosphere the physician carries about him into the sick-chamber, or by the direct application of the virus to the absorbing surfaces with which his hand comes in contact. Many facts and opinions are in favor of each of these modes of transmission."[30] The point is purely logical: the argument from statistical correlation would hold no matter what theory of contagion turned out to be correct, and would survive the replacement of one theory by another.

Holmes's next move is to concentrate on a long list of proven cases in which puerperal fever has followed a single physician from childbed to childbed. Thus, for instance, one Dr. Gooch in the *Philadelphia Medical Journal*: "It is not uncommon for the greater number of cases to occur in the practice of one man, whilst the other practitioners of the neighborhood, who are not more skilful or more busy, meet with few or none. A practitioner opened the body [i.e., performed an autopsy on] of a woman who had died of puerperal fever. . . . A lady whom he delivered a few days afterwards was attacked and died of a similar disease; two more of his lying-in patients, in rapid succession, met with the same fate."[31] Or, even more chillingly, Dr. Gordon of Aberdeen, who, through careful observation in his own locality, had reached the same conclusion fifty years earlier: "I arrived at that certainty in the matter, that I could venture to foretell what women would be affected with the disease, upon hearing by what midwife they were to be delivered, or by what nurse they were to be attended, during their lying-in; and, almost in every instance, my prediction was verified."[32] Holmes would use Gordon's words as an epigraph to the 1855 republication of his essay.

Finally, having provided a list of instances so numerous as to seem almost overwhelming, Holmes rests his argument on the *calcul des probabilités* employed by Paris clinicians from Pinel to Louis. It is something very like the voice of Louis that we hear in Holmes's declaration that he has been dealing not in theories but in established facts. His argument, he says, "allows for the possibility of different modes of conveyance of the destructive principle. It recognizes and supports the belief that a series of cases may originate from a single primitive source which affects each new patient in turn, and especially from cases of Erysipelas. It does not undertake to discuss the theoretical aspect of the subject. . . . Where facts are numerous, and unquestionable, and unequivocal in their significance, theory must follow them as it best may, keeping time with their step, and not go before them, marching to the sound of their own trumpet."[33] In medicine, we recall Louis saying in his *Examen de l'éxamen de M. Broussais,* "what are normally called opinions, or insights, or approaches, belong, properly speaking, to scientific fantasy."

For Holmes, the terrible urgency of the puerperal fever controversy is that, unlike the grandiose speculations with which Broussais had badgered Louis, medical opinions on puerperal fever opposed to his own have an immediate power to kill innocent women. This moral urgency, and not ego or amour propre, explains what might otherwise sound like a tone of preemptive arrogance on Holmes's part: "It signifies nothing that wise and experienced practitioners have sometimes doubted the reality of the danger in question; no man has the right to doubt it any longer. No negative facts, no opposing opinions, be they what they may, or whose they may, can form any answer to the series of cases now within the reach of all who choose to explore the records of medical science."[34] Or, at the end of the essay, even more peremptorily: if "it should be found that the same ominous groups of cases clustering about individual practitioners were observed in a remote country, . . . it would seem incredible that any should be found too prejudiced or indolent to accept the solemn truth knelled into their ears by the funeral bells from both sides of the ocean,—the plain conclusion that the physician and the disease entered, hand in hand, into the chamber of the unsuspecting patient."[35]

The message of Holmes's puerperal fever essay was, in short, that it was not the "destructive principle" carried from bedchamber to bedchamber that was killing new mothers, but bad or faulty logic. The theme would remain central to his writing, both medical and non-medical, for the rest of his career. Yet even within his own group of Boston physicians, his argument met substantial opposition. Dr. Walter Channing, who had been Holmes's own professor of obstetrics at Harvard, and whose report on a number of recent cases of puerperal fever had originally inspired Holmes's own investigations, would subsequently deliver a paper to the Society for Medical Improvement denying that the illness was contagious: "From his own experience he would never hesitate to visit other patients and to take charge of women in labor, when attending puerperal cases as a consulting physician."[36] The medical journal in which

Holmes's essay appeared ceased publication shortly after the essay was printed. Only a short abstract in a more established journal preserved any trace of its original argument.

The 1855 republication of the puerperal fever essay marks Holmes's discovery of his own rhetorical power. Since the journal that printed his original paper folded soon after it appeared, only the short abstract published in the *American Journal of the Medical Sciences* kept Holmes's argument alive. Yet this abstract was enough to attract the attention of some physicians elsewhere, and subsequently an approving mention in a major British publication. It was this last that drew down on Holmes's head the wrath of two of America's most distinguished professors of obstetrics, both of whom sensed a threat to their authority in the transatlantic attention now being paid to his argument. In 1852, Dr. Hugh L. Hodge would refute Holmes's analysis in a lecture published as *On the Non-Contagious Character of Puerperal Fever*. Then, in *Childbed Fevers*, an obstetrics text written in the form of letters to his students at Jefferson Medical College, Dr. Charles D. Meigs derided Holmes's arguments as the "jejeune and fizzenless dreamings" of a sophomoric writer.[37] The puerperal fever issue exploded into a national medical controversy.

By the time Holmes was attacked by Hodge and Meigs, his own situation had altered considerably. Years before, he had written his parents from Paris that the ultimate goal of his studies was not to become a practicing physician but a professor of medicine.[38] He attained his goal early, getting an appointment at Dartmouth Medical School in 1839. Two years later, having gotten married, he resigned his Dartmouth professorship to go briefly into private practice. Then, shortly after having been appointed to a professorship at Harvard in 1847, he gratefully gave up private practice, not least because, as a well-known spokesman for the *méthode expectante*, he found intolerable the pressure to prescribe remedies in which he did not believe. (During his short period of practice, as his case records show, Holmes had felt compelled to prescribe in much the same manner as other physicians.)[39] His decision to reissue his original puerperal fever essay was prompted by a letter from his old Dartmouth colleague Elisha Bartlett, who, wanting to defend Holmes against the attacks of Hodge and Meigs—"How the fungous heads of that Hydra keep sprouting out!" Bartlett cried[40]—asked for offprints. Having long since given away the few copies he had ordered ten years before, Holmes decided to republish the essay as a separate pamphlet.

The writer Hodge and Meigs attacked, therefore, was not the young private physician who had delivered his thoughts on puerperal fever to members of a local medical society, but the Parkman Professor of Anatomy and Physiology at Harvard. He was, in addition, someone who just two years later would earn international acclaim as an author with *The*

Autocrat of the Breakfast Table. It is in *Puerperal Fever as a Private Pestilence*—the new title Holmes gave to the essay when it was now separately published—that he would discover the dynamics of indirect address, involving an amplification of audience through a widening circle of imagined readers, that would make the *Autocrat*, as his contemporary biographer W. S. Kennedy put it, a new kind in literature.[41] For though Dr. Hodge had stayed within the limits of civilized controversy in attacking Holmes, Dr. Meigs had gone farther, pouring ridicule on Holmes for the amusement of the medical students—his "dear young friends," or "dear young gentlemen," as Meigs calls them—addressed in his discourse.

The literary importance of *Puerperal Fever as a Private Pestilence* lies not in the original essay, which Holmes reprinted exactly as it had previously appeared, but in the introductory section in which he takes on the two "widely-known and highly esteemed practitioners, Professors of two of the largest Medical Schools of the Union," who had gone out of their way to attack him. Or rather, its interest lies in the way that his introduction sets up a ratio of address permitting him gradually to shift his gaze outwards past Hodge and Meigs to readers living in a society in which women are going to their graves because such professors as these are excessively enamored of their theories. Holmes's core audience is, ostensibly, the community of practicing physicians addressed in his original essay. But now, thanks to Meigs's own abusive rhetorical tactics, readers have also been made inescapably aware of a larger audience of medical students listening in on any such discourse. This was the occasion of Holmes's experiment with a new rhetorical strategy. For famous professors, as Holmes drily remarks, cannot but influence "in their lectures and printed publications large numbers of young men"[42] who will soon themselves become physicians. And, alas,

> There are some among them who, from youth, or want of training, are easily bewildered and confused in any conflict of opinions into which their studies lead them. They are liable to lose sight of the main question in collateral issues, and to be run away with by suggestive speculations. They confound belief with evidence, often trusting the first because it is expressed with energy, and slighting the latter because it is calm and unimpassioned. They are not satisfied with proof; they cannot believe a point is settled so long as everybody is not silenced.[43]

The essence of Holmes's new strategy, as will be evident from his use of the third person, is to speak not *to* Meigs's "dear young gentlemen," but *about* them to another audience, presumably wiser, more experienced, and less impressionable. This wider audience, to which he addresses his opening remarks, includes "the practitioner, or even the more mature student" who has learned how to draw sound medical conclusions from empirical evidence. Holmes asks the pardon of this wiser, more experienced audience for leading Meig's "dear young gentlemen" through the steps of his original analysis. Given the stakes, it is necessary: "I shall not hesitate to stoop to the most elementary simplicity for the benefit of the younger student. . . . It affords a good opportunity, as it seems to me, of exercising the untrained mind in that medical logic which does not seem to have been either taught or practised in our schools of late, to the extent that might be desired."[44] In a breathtaking display of such medical logic, Holmes reduces his original analysis to a chain of related propositions. Then, using statistics drawn from the Annual Report of the Registrar General in England, he gives the mathematical probability against its being mere coincidence when a single physician in a locality has a substantial series of fatal puerperal cases. It is a billion to one.

As Holmes's address gathers momentum, it becomes clear that its projection of audience also involves a principle of exclusion. Had anyone among his readers been disposed to identify with Meigs's dear young friends at the outset, a reader understands, they have long since departed the scene, or, if they remain, have begun, no doubt somewhat shamefacedly, to shift their allegiance to the group of seasoned practitioners and more mature students to whom Holmes is ostensibly directing the discourse. As Holmes moves forward in his argument, assuming that readers unable to grasp the logic of his analysis are steadily dropping away, he gradually ascends to higher levels of logical inference. On the question of contagion, for instance, Dr. Hodge has attacked Holmes mainly by adducing negative facts—cases in which physicians supposedly carrying puerperal infection delivered women who did *not* come down with the illness. In response Holmes contents himself with quoting a single telling passage from a widely-respected medical textbook: "A man might say, 'I was in the battle of Waterloo, and saw many men around me fall down and die, and it was said that they were struck down by musket-balls; but I know better than that, for I was there all the time, and so were many of my friends, and we were never hit by any musket-balls. Musket-balls, therefore, could not have been the cause of the deaths we witnessed'."[45]

As the ascent to a more universal level of logic begins to leave medical logic as such behind, there is a corresponding universalization of audience, which is more and more taken to include members of a community outside medicine who, listening in on this exchange among physicians, have begun to perceive that they themselves have an important investment in the outcome. Thus, for instance, Dr. Meigs in attacking Holmes had managed to attack the very principle of logical inference itself: "I prefer to attribute them to accident," Meigs had said about deaths of women from puerperal fever, "or to Providence, of which I can form a conception, rather than to a contagion of which I cannot form any clear idea, at least as to this particular malady."[46] Holmes's "sophomoric" arguments, in short, are purely a matter of circumstantial inference. Once again, Holmes answers by quoting another writer. This time, however, the voice is not that of a physician, but of Chief Justice Gibson in the *American Law Journal:*

> "You see a man discharge a gun at another; you see the flash, you hear the report, you see the person fall a lifeless corpse; and you *infer*, from all these circumstances, that there was a ball discharged from the gun, which entered his body and caused his death. . . . But you did not see the ball leave the gun, pass through the air, and enter the body of the slain; and your testimony to the fact of killing is, therefore, only inferential,—in other words, circumstantial. It is *possible* that no ball was in the gun, and we *infer* that there was, only because we cannot account for death on any other supposition."[47]

The horizon of Holmes's discourse has at this point expanded to include all readers with, as he says in the opening paragraphs, "well-constituted and unprejudiced minds."[48] They are locally represented near the end of the essay by the president of a Boston insurance company to whom Holmes takes a set of statistics showing one physician in a neighborhood to have had a series of puerperal fatalities while other doctors delivering babies have had none. Holmes's question: if your company were insuring the life of the next woman to be attended by this doctor, would you demand an extra premium? The president's answer: of course we should demand such a premium, if we should assume the risk at all. Then comes the moment at which this insurance executive, suddenly understanding that Holmes is talking not about hypothetical cases but real women who have died, becomes the angry voice of a outraged community. "I do not choose," says Holmes, "to add the expressions of indignation which the examination of the facts before him called out." He can see from this response alone "that if all the hideous catalogues of cases now accumulated were fully brought to the knowledge of the public, nothing, since the days of Burke and Hare, has raised such a cry of horror as would be shrieked in the ears of the profession."[49]

Drs. Meigs and Hodge make a final appearance in the essay, brought onstage not simply for the benefit of an imaginary audience of doctors and medical students who have been made to face the lethal consequences of lazy or self-interested inference, but, in the distance beyond, a public now made acutely aware of the way that something so apparently innocuous as bad or faulty logic poses a grave danger to the well-being of the community as a whole. Meigs and Hodge are at this point less Holmes's attackers on the puerperal fever issue than the personification of a dangerous professional vanity:

> I only ask the student to read the facts stated by Dr. Condie, as given in my Essay, and say whether or not a man should allow his wife to be attended by a practitioner in whose hands 'scarcely a female that has been delivered for weeks past has escaped an attack,' 'while no instance of the disease has occurred in the patients of any other accoucheur practising in the same district.' If I understand Dr. Meigs and Dr. Hodge, they would not warn the physician or spare the patient under such circumstances. They would 'go on,' if I understand them, not to seven, or seventy, only, but to seventy times seven, if they could find patients. If this is not what they mean, may we respectfully ask them to state what they do mean, to their next classes, in the name of humanity, if not of science![50]

By this point, Holmes is able to gaze through the now-ghostly assemblage of "young students" misled by their professors, through his original audience of unreflective or self-interested medical practitioners, through the body of more enlightened physicians assumed to see the point of Holmes's logic, and even through the professional public locally represented by the president of the insurance company, to a general public by now aware of the momentous stakes involved. The 1855 republication of the puerperal fever essay, in short, marks Holmes's discovery of *double énonciation*, as it is called in formal literary analysis: the mode of indirect address that purports to be speaking to a specific audience—as a trial lawyer, for instance, cross-examines a witness for the benefit of an unaddressed jury—while actually or simultaneously addressing another.[51] The dynamics of *double énonciation* will, beginning with *The Autocrat of the Breakfast Table*, make Holmes the inventor of what W. D. Howells would call the "dramatized essay." Just as Holmes's introductory remarks to the republished puerperal fever essay gradually exclude those who, like Meigs and Hodge, have chosen to persist in their original error, the Breakfast Table trilogy will gradually leave by the wayside those who cannot understand why Holmes and his readers place so great a value on being allowed to discuss "the gravest questions unblamed over our morning coffee-cups or our evening tea-cups."[52]

The end of *Puerperal Fever as a Private Pestilence* is a rhetorical tour de force in which Holmes discovers that the dynamics of *double énonciation* are an entirely legitimate means of simultaneously honoring the two categories of truth he had otherwise learned during his Paris studies to keep separate: those "permanent facts of nature" associated with Louis and the numerical method, which exist in a realm impervious to emotion or sentiment, and that truth of public opinion which, while legitimately and even essentially addressed in civic discourse, is empty or fraudulent in questions resting on empirical evidence. This is what permits Holmes's introduction to the republished version of his essay to assume the status of civic discourse. For the mode of double enunciation that allows him to address its logical and scientific argument to a core group of physicians even while looking outward beyond the horizon of his discourse to a wider audience concludes by dissolving the difference between the two groups in the name of a larger moral principle:

> Let it be remembered that *persons* are nothing in this matter; better that twenty pamphleteers should be silenced, or as many professors unseated, than that one mother's life should be taken. There is no quarrel here between men, but there is deadly incompatibility and exterminating warfare between doctrines. . . . Indifference will not do here; our Journalists and Committees have no right to take up their pages with minute anatomy and tediously detailed cases, while it is a question whether or not the "black death" of child-bed is to be scattered broadcast by the agency of the mother's friend and adviser. Let the men who mould opinions look to it; if there is any voluntary blindness, any interested oversight, any culpable negligence, even, in such a matter, and the facts shall reach the public ear; the pestilence-carrier of the lying-in chamber must look to God for pardon, for man will never forgive him.[53]

The puerperal fever controversy marked Holmes's discovery of a wider public urgently in need of instruction in the principles of sound medical reasoning. This is the audience he would undertake to address in the lyceum lectures subsequently published as *Homeopathy and Its Kindred Delusions*.[54] Since Holmes would later depend on a more consciously popular style of lecturing on literary and cultural topics to meet the expenses of his growing family,[55] it is essential to see that the early lecture on homeopathy had an altogether different motivation. Holmes delivered this lecture at a time when it was still possible to share Ralph Waldo Emerson's hopes for the public lecture as a means of renewing civic spirit in a nation that seemed to be sinking into a crass and ignorant materialism. "I am always haunted with brave dreams of what might be accomplished in the lecture-room," Emerson had written to Carlyle at the beginning of the mid-century craze for lyceum lecturing, "—. . . . I imagine an eloquence of infinite variety,—rich as conversation can be, with anecdote, joke, tragedy, epics and pindarics, argument and confession."[56] "It is the new pulpit," he would tell Carlyle in another letter, "and very much in vogue with my northern countrymen. This winter, in Boston, we shall have . . . two or three every night in the week."[57]

Emerson was responsible for Holmes's career as a lyceum lecturer. At the famous Harvard Phi Beta Kappa Society meeting at which Emerson delivered "The American Scholar," Holmes had read a poem composed for the same occasion. Impressed by Holmes's wit and polish in public performance, Emerson then suggested him as a lyceum lecturer. The spirit in which he did so is caught in another of his letters to Carlyle: "There are in this country so few scholars, that the services of each studious person are needed to do what he can for the circulation of thoughts, to the end of making some counterweight to the money force."[58] The sense of civic purpose in Emerson's remark is a key to the way Holmes would subsequently use medicine as what might be called an encrypted mode of civic discourse. For medicine is at once entirely democratic— every citizen has a body, with ills and pains that are no respecters of wealth or rank or status—and at the same time based on the authority of hard-won specialized knowledge. To Holmes, just back from Paris, the notion that rigorous training was the only legitimate source of medical authority seemed, in a climate of medical charlatanism increasingly given to justifying itself in the language of Jacksonian democracy—what I shall mean by the term "Jacksonian medicine"—to carry important civic implications.

In homeopathy, Holmes found a ready example of the ways even educated and thoughtful citizens could show themselves eager to embrace illogical claims. His presentation begins not with homeopathy itself but medical superstitions from the credulous past: the *unguentum armarium*, for instance, a miraculous ointment that in the time of Bacon and Shakespeare was imagined to have worked its cures by being rubbed not on the soldier's wound, but on the weapon that caused it. Or, at the turn of the nineteenth century, the brief and hilarious career of Perkins's metallic tractors, short implements of iron and brass which were to be drawn slowly over the injured portion of the body—the inspiration was obviously the newly-discovered phenomenon of Galvinism—devised by an enterprising Connecticut Yankee and advertised in England with glowing testimonials from Dukes, Bishops, and members of the Royal Family. The *unguentum armarium* was an obscure bit of remote medical history, and Perkins's metallic tractors a medical fad remembered only by older people in New England. Yet the arguments used to support both, Holmes sets about showing, were the same as those now being used to support homeopathy.

Homeopathy and Its Kindred Delusions is a series of lessons in elementary logical reasoning. Homeopathy was invented by Samuel Hahnemann, a German physician whose *Organon of the Healing Art*, published in 1810, claimed to have overturned all previous medical systems in the name of several great discoveries. Consider Holmes's treatment of one of them, the doctrine of minute or infinitesimal dosage. Such standard remedies as quinine were given an honorable place in the homeopathic pharmacopeia. But for homeopathy, the secret of their efficacy lay entirely in the preparation. A grain of quinine, for instance, is to be mixed with the third part of a hundred grains of sugar of milk (lactose), then rubbed for six minutes in an unglazed vessel. Holmes goes on: "Four minutes are then to be devoted to scraping the powder into a heap, and the second third of the hundred grains of sugar of milk to be added. Then they are to be stirred an instant and rubbed six minutes,—again to be scraped together four minutes and forcibly rubbed six; once more scraped together for four minutes, when the last third of the hundred grains of sugar of milk is to be added and mingled by stirring with the spatula; six minutes of forcible rubbing, four of scraping together, and six more (positively the last six) of rubbing, finish this part of the process."[59]

The rubbing and scraping is followed by successive dilutions in alcohol, in which the substance is shaken, a drop removed and added to another quantity of pure alcohol, shaken again—Holmes solemnly quotes Hahnemann: "A long experience and multiplied observations upon the sick lead me within the last few years to prefer giving only two shakes to medicinal liquids, whereas I formerly used to give ten"[60]—a drop removed and added to more alcohol, and so on. The dosage thus yielded is almost literally infinitesimal. Suppose, Holmes says, that one were to achieve the same degree of dilution simply by *adding* alcohol to the first measure: "For the fourth dilution it would take . . . more than 1,000 gallons, and so on to the ninth dilution, which would take ten billion gallons," which the Italian scientist who made these calculations "computed would fill the basin of Lake Agnano, a body of water two miles in circumference. . . . By the time the seventeenth degree of dilution should be reached, the alcohol required would equal in quantity the waters of ten thousand Adriatic seas."[61] The homeopath is proposing, in short, something like the modern equivalent of suggesting that a person cure a headache by dropping an aspirin in Lake Superior and then drinking a cup of its water.

Setting aside the other logical absurdities on which the homeopathic system is based—the principle, for instance, of *similia similibus curantur*, or idea that diseases are cured by substances that cause the same symptoms in healthy individuals—the doctrine of infinitesimal doses alone might seem to be enough to discredit its claims. But, as Holmes understands, such systems are usually supported, as the claims for Perkins's metallic tractors were tacitly supported by a popular awareness of Galvinism, by false analogy with some valid principle of medical knowledge. In the case of homeopathy, the borrowed validity is coming from Jenner's discovery of vaccination. Ask a homeopathist about the power of his infinitesimal doses, says Holmes,

and he will answer by referring to the effects produced by a very minute portion of vaccine matter. . . . But the vaccine matter is one of those substances called *morbid poisons*, of which it is a peculiar character to multiply themselves, when introduced into the system, as a seed does in the soil. Therefore the hundredth part of a grain of the vaccine matter, if no more than this is employed, soon increases in quantity, until, in the course of about a week, it is a grain or more, and can be removed in considerable drops. . . . The thoughtlessness which can allow an inference to be extended from a product of disease possessing this susceptibility of multiplication when conveyed into the living body, to substances of inorganic origin, such as silex or sulphur, would be capable of arguing that a pebble may produce a mountain, because an acorn can become a forest.[62]

Yet Holmes's deeper point is that homeopathy is sustained by the same false reasoning found in many other forms of medical error, including the bleeding, purging, drugging practice of many regularly-educated American physicians. The *vis medicatrix naturae* is what cures every patient who gets well. The physician's lie—or delusion, if it springs from honest self-deception—is to claim that his remedies brought about the cure. Nobody doubts, as Holmes points out, that *some* patients get well under every regimen. Indeed, ninety in a hundred would probably recover, "sooner or later, with more or less difficulty, provided nothing were done to interfere seriously with the efforts of nature." Now suppose that a physician were to have given these same hundred patients pills made of sugar or starch. There must, in such a case, "be a considerable number of coincidences between the relief of the patient and the administration of the remedy. It is altogether probable that there will happen two or three *very striking* coincidences . . . in which it would seem evident that the medicine produced the relief, though it had . . . nothing to do with it." [63] The doctor who mistakenly or duplicitously claims credit for the cure is, in Holmes's eyes, simply repeating the entire history of medicine from Galen to the present day.

A crucial question is why Holmes made homeopathy his target, rather than the numerous forms of popular charlatanism flourishing in Jacksonian America. As we have seen, he campaigned within his own profession for the *médecine expectante* associated with Paris medicine, denouncing the bleeding, purging, drugging practice of regular physicians as being based on the same error as homeopathy. "The inveterate logical errors to which physicians have always been subject," he remarks in a later essay—and here he means regularly educated physicians as much as homeopaths—have remained the same, chief among them being "the mode of inference *per enumerationem simplicem,* in scholastic phrase: that is, counting only their favorable cases." Louis's "numerical system," he declares, "is the best corrective of this error."[64] Homeopathy, moreover, with its European antecedents, its journals and its diplomas and professional organizations, aimed for at least the appearance of medical respectability. A much more serious threat to the genuine medical authority for which Holmes always argued, based on knowledge of "the natural progress of a malady, of its ordinary duration, of its various modes of terminating,"[65] would seem to have been posed by the rapidly multiplying varieties of popular medicine given to justifying their claims in the language of Jacksonian democracy.

The most celebrated was Thomsonian botanical practice. It was based on the theories of Samuel Thomson, a rural New Hampshire practitioner who took it upon himself to proclaim the truth of a now neglected Greek medicine—the elements making up the human body really were, he decided, earth, air, fire and water—and a notion of humoral balance running back through the Brunonian system of "sthenic" and "asthenic" disorders to Galen and Hippocrates. Thomson's major discovery was that the balance constituting health was a result of "natural heat" in the body. Most disorders were caused by excessive cold. Fever, an ally of the physician, was caused by obstructed perspiration, for which the remedies were emetics and purges, to clear the system and restore the natural balance. Thomson's *New Guide to Health* was based on one further principle destined to give his system enormous popular appeal. The substances used to restore balance should be botanical or vegetable remedies familiar in the centuries before a class of privileged individuals had conspired to make medicine into a mystery and professional education into a means of duping ordinary people.

The roots of Thomsonian medicine went back ultimately to the radical religious movements of the English Interregnum, where sects like the Levelers and the Fifth Monarchy Men had been prompt to denounce any pretensions to specialized learning as violations of an original and divinely-ordained equality. In the eighteenth century, John Wesley, the moving spirit of Methodism and author of the popular medical guide *Primitive Physick,* would similarly denounce professional medicine as a conspiracy of spurious "learning." Medicine had once been simple, but then it had become, said Wesley, a matter of textbooks and Latin names, "till at length Physick became an abstruse Science, quite out of the Reach of Ordinary men."[66] In nineteenth-century America, Samuel Thomson would use the newer political vocabulary of Jacksonian democracy to similarly anathematize anyone claiming education as a basis of special authority:

Fellow citizens . . . you have plenty of good men among you, who are as capable as those who have studied law, physick, or divinity, and are much safer to be trusted; they will feel the same interest with you . . . and not make laws for the benefit of the few, to the injury of the whole. The influence of the professional gentlemen is now very great in the public councils. . . . Many of the gentlemen alluded to, profess a great deal of republicanism; this is all a false pretence, for it is as much impossible that one of the learned professions can be a republican, as it is for ice to produce heat. The very nature of their situation, and the relation in which they stand to the rest of society forbids it. They are a privileged class of men, and their existence as such depends entirely upon their being looked up to as a superior order and are in fact as complete an aristocracy as exists in any part of the world.[67]

A great part of Thomson's popular appeal had to do with his polemic against the "grammar doctors" who read Latin and Greek. Holmes, with his love of reading the medical texts of earlier ages, might in this instance have been Thomson's specific target. "Shall I ever forget that rainy day in Lyons," Holmes will say in his wonderful essay on medical libraries, "that dingy bookshop, where I found the Aëtius, long missing from my *Artis Medicæ Principes?*"[68] But Greek and Latin names, Thomson had said many years before, as if to anticipate such unapologetic pleasure in arcane learning, never set a fractured leg, dressed a wound, or cured a dropsy. As one Thomsonian practitioner impatiently remarked, such learning was "useless rubbish to more than seven-eighths of us."[69] As important, medical authority did not necessarily involve an ability to read and write. Peruvian natives had discovered the virtue of cinchona bark against malaria, after all, and dairy maids had known about the immunizing properties of cowpox before Jenner. "The scientific faculty are more indebted to the illiterate for rudimental knowledge," declared the Thomsonian polemicist Thomas Hersey, ". . . than the illiterate are to all the learned labors of the world."[70]

As Holmes himself would ruefully recognize, another part of the Thomsonians' popular appeal came from their denunciation of the bleeding and "mineral poisons" authorized by Rush's system of heroic practice, precisely the same battle Holmes was himself fighting under the standard of the *méthode expectante*. "The great difficulty I have had to encounter in removing the complaints which my patients laboured under," said Thomson in his *New Guide to Health*, "has been to clear the system of mercury, nitre, or opium." Doctors administer these substances "under the specious pretense of great skill and art," he adds, but that pretense "will not blind the people, if they would examine and think for themselves, instead of believing that every thing said or done by a learned man must be right."[71] In 1849, the editor of the Jacksonian *United States Magazine, and Democratic Review* would quote the Enlightenment philosopher D'Alembert to make the same point: "Nature is fighting with disease; a blind man armed with a club,—that is, the physician—comes to settle the difference. . . . When he cannot accomplish this, he lifts his club and strikes at random. If he strikes the disease, he kills the disease; if he strikes nature, he kills the patient."[72]

In the immediate background of Thomsonian botanical practice lurked even more radical varieties of Jacksonian medicine, similarly based on the claim that professional knowledge was a hoax devised by a privileged class to exploit ordinary people. A good example is Daniel H. Whitney's *The Family Physician: or Every Man His Own Doctor*, a complete system of medicine intended to liberate citizens in a democracy from the tyranny of regular physicians. For the principles of the healing art, Whitney explains, are no more mysterious than those of any ordinary trade. If readers were willing to take a few hours to learn them, "they would be no more under the necessity of sending for a physician to tell them what kind, and how much medicine they must take . . . than they are now of sending for the butcher or the baker, to determine the kind and quantity of food they should eat, and the proper time of using it; or of calling on the tailor for instructions for putting on their woolens." In the materia medica, especially, "physicians have ever found a tower impregnable to the mass of the people, and which they have rendered inaccessible by entrenching it around with difficult terms of their own invention."[73]

The Family Physician goes beyond most popular manuals of Jacksonian medicine, however, in giving simple step-by-step instructions for performing major surgery at home using common household implements. For instance, Whitney cheerfully explains, "any man of common dexterity and firmness of nerve, can cut off a limb, as safely as a surgeon."[74] The necessary instruments can be found around the house: for the bone saw, a carpenter's saw; for the amputating knife, "a carving or other large knife, with a smooth, sharp, and straight blade"; for the scalpel, a penknife; for the dressing, "a piece of linen large enough to cover the end of the stump, spread with simple ointment or lard."[75] Amputation of, say, the arm, is a simple enough procedure: "Let one support the lower end of the arm, and . . . another draw up the skin. Now with the large knife make one cut straight around the limb through the skin and fat only. Then with the small knife separate as much of the skin from the flesh above the cut as will form a flap to cover the face of the stump, turn this back, and let it be held by an assistant. With the large knife make a second incision round the arm and down to the bone, as close as you can to the skin you have turned back, taking care not to cut it."[76]

Given the strong affinities between Thomsonian medicine and Jacksonian ideology in politics, it was perhaps inevitable that denunciation of "grammar doctors" would lead to a movement to abolish medical licensing. Thomson himself demanded a repeal of legislation regulating medical practice. The movement won a significant victory in New York in 1844, in which medical licensing laws were repealed in response to a popular petition. "The people of this state have been bled long enough in their bodies and their pockets," thundered one New York legislator.[77] "Men cannot be legislated out of one religion and into another," said the committee report that led to the repeal. "Nor can the Legislature thrust calomel and mercury down a man's throat while he wills to take only cayenne or lobelia."[78] In Ohio, Thomsonians described licensing as bestowing on regularly-educated physicians nothing less than the outrageous "legal privilege of sporting, tampering and speculating with the health, life and property of our citizens."[79] Opposition to a bill granting a charter to a Thomsonian school, one prominent Ohio politician darkly warned, would be taken by voters as "a mark of an aristocratical and monopolizing disposition that should have no place in an American bosom."[80]

A dozen passages might be lifted out of Holmes's writings that would, in the absence of further information, seem to be directed at precisely this sort of Jacksonian appeal to popular opinion. For such appeals, as he once says, are clearly based on "an attempt to show the insignificance of all existing medical knowledge," to show that regular medical practice is "attended with the most positively injurious effects," and that "by it acute diseases are aggravated, and chronic diseases rendered incurable."[81] "These and similar accusations, so often brought up against the Medical Profession," he says elsewhere, "are only one mode in which is manifested a spirit of opposition not merely to medical science, but to all science, and to all sound knowledge. It is a spirit which neither understands itself nor the object at which it is aiming." It purports to prove, he goes on, "that the persons who have passed their lives in the study of a branch of knowledge the very essence of which must always consist in long and accurate observation, are less competent to judge of new doctrines in their own department than the rest of the community. It belongs to the clown in society, the destructive in politics, and the rogue in practice."[82]

Yet these passages occur not in some polemic against Jacksonian medicine, but in *Homeopathy and Its Kindred Delusions*, again raising the question of why Holmes chose a minor and relatively harmless form of charlatanism—infinitesimal doses as opposed to the bold amputation of a neighbor's arm at the kitchen table—as his target. In standard histories of American medicine, the answer tends to be given in terms of market competition. "Homeopathy," explains Martin Kaufman, "was more of a threat to the medical profession than Thomsonianism had been. In the first place, . . . many homeopaths were recruited from the regular profession. . . . Nor were its practitioners the uneducated backwoodsmen attracted to Thomsonianism; rather, they were well-educated individuals who had discarded their original methods because of their inadequacy."[83] Contemporary sources amply support such a view. "Many of the learned, accomplished, and, what is more to the purpose, the *wealthy*," lamented one regularly-educated physician in the *Boston Medical and Surgical Journal* in 1844, "have an unconquerable aversion to taking nauseous and bitter medicines. . . . Hence a homeopathist is preferred by such."[84]

In Holmes's case, such an interpretation poses several major problems. The first is that he had himself campaigned against the nauseous and bitter medicines given by regular practitioners virtually since his return from Paris. Indeed, the one concession he would always make to homeopathy was that its harmless remedies and infinitesimal doses had the great virtue of turning patients against drugs like calomel and tartar emetic, as well as against the copious bleeding authorized by Rush's heroic practice. A second problem is that Holmes's language, as when he associates homeopathy with the clown in society or the destructive in politics, seems more obviously suited to Thomson's botanical practice and Whitney's *The Family Physician* than to the learned and accomplished souls mentioned by the writer in the *Boston Medical and Surgical Journal*. These are the paradoxes that permit us to see that Holmes, in talking about clowns and rogues and quacks, or in arguing that what threatens a community is not doctrines like homeopathy but the "ignorance, error, or deception"[85] that permits them to flourish, is talking not about social classes or party politics but about the increasing tyranny of an ignorant majority in his own nineteenth-century America.

Homeopathy and Its Kindred Delusions thus demands to be read as an early demonstration of the way Holmes would always conceive his own purpose as a writer: as an attempt to alter the thinking of a minority that he saw as having a regenerative power in a republic otherwise sinking into indiscriminate populism. It is by surrendering to the market pressures Emerson calls the "money force," or by taking seriously Jacksonian railing against "aristocratical" conspiracies, that one becomes destructive in politics or a clown in society, whether one has been born on Beacon Hill or in the backwoods of Kentucky. The minority that resists such pressures has a power out of proportion to its numbers, in turn, because it is allied with a larger order of truth, or what Holmes once calls "the permanent facts of nature."[86] This is the special sense in which medical truth—Bichat's pathological correlations, for instance, or Laennec's victory over Broussais, based on the demonstrable truth of stethoscopic results—will always serve as Holmes's primary example of such an order. It is in one of his medical essays that Holmes issues what may be taken as the manifesto of his entire literary career:

This Republic is the chosen home of *minorities*, of the less power in the presence of the greater. It is a common error to speak of our distinction as consisting in the rule of the majority. Majorities, the greater material powers, have always ruled before. The history of most countries has been that of majorities,—mounted majorities, clad in iron, armed with death, treading down the tenfold more numerous minorities. In the old civilizations they root themselves in the soil; men must live in their shadow or cut them down. With us the majority is only the flower of the passing noon, and the minority is the bud which may open in the next morning's sun. We must be tolerant, for the thought which stammers on a single tongue today may organize itself in the growing consciousness of the time, and come back to us like the multitudinous waves of the ocean on the morrow.[87]

The minority Holmes is talking about is the same class of educated and thoughtful souls that Matthew Arnold, using a language alive with Biblical resonance, had called the saving remnant.[88] In an age driven by crass materialism and indiscriminate populism, Holmes would always place his own hopes for its redemption in bringing this saving remnant to a consciousness of its own power to resist error and establish truth. As in his medical essays he projected as his true audience a body of learned physicians opposed to ignorance and popular error, so in the Breakfast Table books would Holmes work to summon into existence a moral and intellectual minority holding the promise of civic regeneration in the new world of Jacksonian ideology. "Our American atmosphere," he remarks in one essay, "is vocal with the flippant loquacity of half knowledge. We must accept whatever good can be got out of it, and keep it under as we do sorrel and mullein and witch grass, by enriching the soil, and sowing good seed in plenty; by good teaching and good books, rather than wasting our time in talking against it."[89] Holmes's own attempt to sow good seed in the wider world beyond medicine would begin in the pages of the *Atlantic Monthly* in the fall of 1857, with the appearance of the first installment of *The Autocrat of the Breakfast Table.*

CHAPTER FIVE

Religio Medici

"*F*aith," said Sainte-Beuve in that passage Holmes found remarkable enough to copy into his personal notebook, "has disappeared. Science, let people say what they will, has destroyed it." On both sides of the Atlantic, Victorian religious anxiety was experienced in Sainte-Beuve's terms, with science taken as the bleak revelation of a dead universe in which the only ultimate laws are those of physics and chemistry. "Are we only helpless particles," asked Charles Kingsley, "at best separate parts of the wheels of a vast machine, which will use us till it has worn us away, and ground us to powder? Are our bodies—and if so, why not our souls?—the puppets, yea the creatures of necessary circumstances?"[1] The despair to which this bleak picture led is nowhere better caught than in an autobiographical passage by Frederick Robertson: "It is an awful hour—let him who has passed through it say how awful—when this life has lost its meaning, and seems shrivelled into a span; when the grave appears to be the end of all, human goodness nothing but a name, and the sky above this universe a dead expanse, black with the void from which God himself has disappeared."[2] This is the background against which Holmes, wholly aware of its implications for himself as a scientifically-trained physician, would pick up his pen to compose the first number of *The Autocrat of the Breakfast Table*.

In *The Autocrat*, the speaker holding forth at the breakfast table does not yet identify himself as a physician, although we always understand that he spent several years in Paris pursuing studies that sound very much like medical training. In *The Professor at the Breakfast Table*, the second volume of the series, the speaker is a teacher at a well-known medical school, fully in touch with the latest discoveries of scientific medicine. In *The Poet at the Breakfast Table*, the final volume, the Professor's role as a spokesman for modern science is taken over by one of the boarders, the learned polymath called the Master, wholly familiar with Lyell's geology and Darwin's evolutionary theory and Pasteur's germ theory of disease. It is the Master who shows a easy and untroubled familiarity with the materialism of works which, like Cabanis's *Traité du physique et du moral de l'homme*, had inspired the Paris medical revolution. For the Master had passed a good deal of his youth, as he once discloses, among "the inner circle of rationalists, who believed in the persistence of Force, and the identity of alimentary substances with virtue, and were reconstructing the universe on this basis, with absolute exclusion of all Supernumeries."[3]

From the *Autocrat of the Breakfast Table* onwards, Holmes would always oppose to such materialist doctrines a metaphysics of consciousness that imposed strict limits on the claims of scientific truth. This is the metaphysics we glimpse at those moments in Holmes's medical essays where, normally addressing an audience of fellow physicians, he need not fear being accused of blasphemy for treating the physical sciences as, in effect, the modern form of divine revelation:

> Once more, we cannot fail to see that just as astrology has given place to astronomy, so theology, the science of Him whom by searching no man can find out, is fast being replaced by what we may not improperly called theonomy, or the science of the laws according to which the Creator acts. And since these laws find their fullest manifestations for us, at least, in rational human natures, the study of anthropology is largely replacing that of scholastic divinity. We must contemplate our Maker indirectly in human attributes as we talk of Him in human parts of speech. And this gives a sacredness to the study of man in his physical, mental, moral, social, and religious nature.[4]

In the Breakfast Table trilogy, addressed to the more miscellaneous readership of the *Atlantic*, Holmes would always feel a need to be careful of the sensibility of those still subject to the imperatives of an older religious orthodoxy. His metaphysics of consciousness, accordingly, would be communicated mainly as a matter of voice and moral perspective, revealed in the way the Autocrat talks about a myriad of topics apparently unrelated to science or religion. Yet the flow of conversation will always move towards that conception of science that Holmes had brought back from his Paris medical studies, and that has only been strengthened by his subsequent medical and scientific reading. Whenever science or religion explicitly arise as topics in the trilogy, two related points may be glimpsed just beneath the surface of the discourse: (1) science, whose triumph in the modern age has been seen by souls like Sainte-Beuve to have annihilated the possibility of religious belief, is, as much as art or literature, a creation of human consciousness, and (2) the physical sciences, justly celebrated for their power to explain the workings of a blind material universe, have no power whatever to explain the phenomenon of consciousness.

In a very general sense, Holmes's views on the relation between mind and external reality are Kantian. "The forms or conditions of Time and Space," the Autocrat reminds his readers, "as Kant will tell you, are nothing in themselves,—only our way of looking at things."[5] Yet the great point of Kant's philosophy, that time, space, and causality are simply an empty grid that the mind imposes on the raw flux of experience, does not stress the principle to which Holmes meant his Breakfast Table books to serve as permanent testimony. This is the point that any attempt by consciousness to examine its own nature—the attempt, as one might say, to discover some vantage point outside itself from which it could be examined—involves what in logic is called an infinite regress. It is an ancient philosophical paradox: whenever I examine the contents of my own mind, the "I" of my ordinary experience must ascend to an as-yet-unexamined vantage point separate from what I am examining. To try to examine *that* vantage point I must ascend to another—and so on, outwards to infinity. Holmes's originality as a writer lies in having taken this paradox as setting a strict limit to the questions that may be intelligibly asked about God, man, and nature.

If rational consciousness must for purely logical reasons remain mysterious, in short, and if scientific theories are always a product of rational consciousness, then Sainte-Beuve's despairing vision of a war between science and religion is based on a mistake. Science, Holmes will say in *The Professor at the Breakfast Table*, "in other words, knowledge,—is not the enemy of religion; for, if so, then religion would mean ignorance."[6] So it is that Holmes will be able to provide readers of the Breakfast Table trilogy with a view of nineteenth-century science—the unimaginable stretches of geological time opened up by Lyell's *Principles of Geology*, the nebular hypothesis in astronomy, the physiological basis of health and disease as studied by his teachers at the École de Médecine—as a demonstration that human consciousness does not ultimately belong to that blind whirl of atoms and molecules that is the domain of the physical sciences:

> A man that knows men, in the street, at their work, human nature in its shirt-sleeves, . . . above all, who has found out, by living into the pith and core of life, that all the Deity which can be folded up between the sheets of any human book is to the Deity of the firmament, of the strata, of the hot aortic flood of human life, of this infinite, instantaneous consciousness in which the soul's being consists,—an incandescent point in the filament connecting the negative pole of a past eternity with the positive pole of an eternity that is to come . . . gets some things into his head he might not find in the index of his "Body of Divinity."[7]

There is a further paradox. Holmes's metaphysics also assumes that the originary or primordial status of rational consciousness is not something that could be established by argument, since consciousness—like language, logic, and thought itself— must always be presupposed before argument can begin. This is why Holmes's turn to literary expression in the Breakfast Table books carries so important a burden of philosophical implication. For the originary power of consciousness has never been denied in literary works: Homer and Virgil and Shakespeare live on, generations have agreed to say, because out of language their genius created worlds. The Breakfast Table books, written in a stream-of-consciousness style that continuously dramatizes that infinite, instantaneous consciousness in which the soul's being consists, amount to a single extended demonstration that language, logic, and thought, and not the dead universe of the physical sciences, are the true home of human consciousness. The flow of his thoughts, Holmes will once remark in *The Poet at the Breakfast Table*, has been as sinuous as the Connecticut River, which he has just been describing, and "from which I please myself with thinking that I have learned to wind without fretting against the shore, or forgetting where I am flowing."[8]

The stream-of-consciousness style of the Breakfast Table books took over in more or less direct terms the extraordinary conversational powers for which Holmes had been remarked since his youth. Holmes, like Samuel Johnson in eighteenth-century England or Oscar Wilde in his own time, was one of those rare souls who can only be described as a genius in conversation.[9] As early as 1839, for instance, when both he and Holmes were on the faculty of Dartmouth Medical School, Elisha Bartlett would describe these to his friend Dr. John Orne Green: "His attainments in medical science are extensive and accurate, and his intellectual endowments are extraordinary. His mind is quick as lightning and sharp as a razor. His conversational powers are absolutely wonderful. . . . His talk at table is all spontaneous, unpremeditated, and he pours himself forth—words and thoughts—in a perfect torrent. His wit and humour are quite lost in the prodigal exuberance of his thoughts and language."[10] The major distinction is that Holmes will always make a point of speaking in the Breakfast Table books, as he did not in ordinary conversation, as the representative voice of Boston culture.

The moral and intellectual drama of the Breakfast Table series derives from Holmes's sense of Boston as a besieged citadel of civic values in a nation increasingly coming under the domination of Jacksonian democracy, an indiscriminate populism bent on doing away with all distinctions based on learning, intelligence, or sense of civic responsibility. The most controversial parts of the *Autocrat* were those where the speaker opts for cultural background as a measure of social worth. "The right of strict social discrimination of all things and persons," the Autocrat says in the opening pages, is "one of the most precious republican privileges. I take the liberty to exercise it when I say that, *other things being equal,* in most relations of life I prefer a man of family."[11] What does he mean by a man of family? The answer is self-mockingly given, as though such a question could be answered by a mere catalogue of household furnishings: ancestral portraits by Smibert and Copley, family silver, claw-footed chairs and black mahogany tables, stately upright cabinets to hold old books—"Pope, original edition, 15 volumes, London, 1717. Barrow on the lower shelves in folio. Tillotson on the upper, in a little dark platoon of octodecimos"[12]—but the point is entirely serious.

The values to which the Autocrat is declaring allegiance at such moments belong to classical republican political theory, an ancient language of the polity going back to Aristotle's *Politics* and widely spoken in both England and America in the period leading up to the Revolutionary War.[13] The particular value he associates with family or cultural circumstance was in the classical republican idiom called *virtus,* always directly translated as "virtue" in eighteenth-century writing: the ability on the part of citizens to put the well-being of the polity over private or individual self-interest. To those raised in the ethos of New England Federalism, the antithesis of civic virtue was the crude economic individualism they associated with the triumph of Jacksonian democracy in the 1830s. The Autocrat's point is not that those born into an established lineage are in any natural sense superior to those who are not—a notion that Holmes detested, especially as embodied in the British system of inherited or titled privilege—but simply that circumstances favor their being the bearers of certain essential civic values:

> One may, it is true, have all the antecedents I have spoken of, and yet be a boor or a shabby fellow. One may have none of them, and yet be fit for councils or courts. Then let them change places. Our social arrangement has this great beauty, that its strata shift up and down as they change specific gravity, without being clogged by layers of prescription. But I still insist on my democratic liberty of choice, and I go for the man with the gallery of family portraits against the one with the twenty-five-cent daguerreotype, unless I find out that the last is the better of the two.[14]

In the immediate background of the Autocrat's dictum is the New England Federalism that had always seen the greatest threat to the hard-won gains of the Revolution—the epochal struggle that had preserved the American colonies, in all their republican simplicity, from the corruption of an older European civilization[15]—in a money or market society intent on demolishing an ancient structure of civic values based on moral and intellectual character. "The single passion that engrosses us," the great Boston Federalist Fisher Ames had said in the days of the early republic, "the only avenue to consideration and importance in our society, is the accumulation of property; our inclinations cling to gold, and are bedded in it, as deeply as that precious ore in the mines."[16] A few years later, William Ellery Channing would lament "the mournful effects of the infinite, intense thirst for gain and accumulation" in the young American republic. In time, he added with a brave hopefulness, Americans may yet come to realize "that money is not the supreme end of the social compact, that republican institutions in particular have liberty and improvement and the development of human nature for their objects."[17]

Before he began the Breakfast Table series, as we have seen, Holmes's own opposition to Jacksonian ideology was expressed in his campaign against medical quackery, with Boston representing not simply the *méthode expectante* but an idea of medical authority based on rigorous training and clinical experience. Physicians like Holmes were always attacked by their more extreme opponents in the idiom of indiscriminate populism associated with Jacksonian democracy. Regularly-educated physicians, we recall the botanical practitioner Samuel Thomson saying, "are a privileged class of men" whose privilege "depends entirely upon their being looked up to as a superior order." They are, he added, "as complete an aristocracy as exists in any part of the world."[18] Thomson's specific target was American doctors who held the M.D. Had he been aiming at physicians like Henry Bowditch, Jr., Mason Warren, and Oliver Wendell Holmes, whose credentials included not simply the Harvard M.D. but several years of Paris medical training, he would doubtless have used terms still more violent. This is the perspective that Holmes, as we may also recall, dismissed as belonging to "the clown in society, the destructive in politics, and the rogue in practice."

In the *Autocrat of the Breakfast Table*, Holmes's personal opposition to Jacksonian medicine is transposed into a grand symbolic opposition between Boston and Jacksonian America. In particular, the *Autocrat* is a response to the America controversially portrayed some years earlier in Frances Trollope's *Domestic Manners of the Americans*, with its whisky-swilling, tobacco-spitting population given to loud boasting about the glories of American democracy. For Mrs. Trollope, who had chosen the American boarding house as the very symbol of an entire society dissolving into little more than a random conglomeration of solitary souls,[19] had been especially struck by the tendency of Jacksonian democracy to reduce life to a level of mere animal existence. "They eat with the greatest possible rapidity," she says wonderingly about one such boarding house, "and in total silence."[20] Elsewhere, she and her female companions are reduced to wordless amazement by "the total want of all the usual courtesies of the table, the voracious rapidity with which viands were seized and devoured, . . . the loathsome spitting, from the contamination of which it was absolutely impossible to protect our dresses; the frightful manner of feeding with their knives, till the whole blade seemed to enter the mouth; and the still more frightful manner of cleaning the teeth afterwards with a pocket knife."[21]

To Mrs. Trollope's image of Jacksonian backwoods democracy, the Breakfast Table trilogy opposes the image of a Boston blessed with a long tradition of publicly-supported education—"Boston is a happy place to live in," the distinguished Harvard scholar George Ticknor had said, "because all the people are educated"[22]—with writers and philosophers like Emerson and Thoreau and Hawthorne and Holmes—"These expressed with ripened fulness," William Dean Howells would later say, looking back on the Boston in which he had arrived as a young man, "a civilization conceived in faith and brought forth in good works"[23]—and with a sense of civic purpose virtually unknown in the vast hinterlands of Jacksonian democracy. This was the classical republican value of *virtus* as members of old Boston families associated it with the Puritan origins of their own New England society. It was the "stern republicanism" of the Puritan fathers, declared Edward Warren, son and biographer of Holmes's teacher John Collins Warren, that insisted "that the descendant of a duke should be entitled to no higher honor than the descendant of the meanest peasant. Patriotism, the general good of the community, next to God, was to be the sole object of worship."[24]

Yet the actual Boston in which Holmes dwelt was, as he conceived it, still very far from being an ideal society. Boston was burdened, in the first place, by the inheritance of the New England Calvinism that in the Breakfast Table books will always be portrayed as the gloomy antithesis of all that is genuinely liberating in modern thought. This was the New England theology of the Puritan fathers and Jonathan Edwards, based on the worship of a vengeful Old Testament deity who created numberless human beings doomed to spend an eternity in the torments of a Hell to which, according to Calvin's doctrine of predestination, they had been condemned even before their birth. The whole point of Edwards's theology, Holmes would grimly observe, had been to "burn these horrors into the souls of men": "The body is to possess the most exquisite sensibilities, it is to be pervaded in every fibre and particle by the fire, and the fire is to be such that our lime-kilns and iron-furnaces would be refrigerators in comparison with the mildest of the torture-chambers. Here the great majority of mankind are to pass the days and nights . . . of a sleepless eternity."[25]

In the second place, the Boston intellectual culture in whose name the Autocrat speaks has been viewed, fairly or unfairly, as limited and provincial, or, worse, as merely a second-hand imitation of British civilization. "The Bostonian," complained W. S. Kennedy, "is simply an Americanized Englishman." "As the Englishman is the physical bully of the world, so the Bostonian is the aesthetic and intellectual bully of America": "underneath the high polish of consummate manners," Kennedy maintained, lurks "the stony glare of self-aggrandizement, the icy complacency of ancestral pride (*odi profanum vulgus*), the *de haut en bas* air of an intellectual and social aristocracy well ballasted by the weighty annals of the past."[26] The charge is rooted in political antagonisms going back to the earliest days of the American republic, when such New England Federalists as John Adams and Fisher Ames had identified strongly with Great Britain in her long and lonely struggle against Napoleon, while Thomas Jefferson and the radical democrats of William Duane's *Aurora*, undismayed by the bloody reign of Robespierre and the Jacobin party, continued just as strongly to identify themselves with revolutionary France.[27]

This is a polarity Holmes sets out to reverse in the *Autocrat* by creating an idealized Boston whose cosmopolitan values will unexpectedly come to be associated with French rather than British culture. In doing so, he was giving public currency to a perception that one encounters again and again in memoirs of the Boston medical students who were with him in Paris. Thus, for instance, Howard Payson Arnold, fresh from a reading of the Paris journals of Holmes's friend Mason Warren: "under every aspect, Paris stood out in vivid contrast with Boston, whose Puritanical leaven and well-worn categorical ruts" seemed stultifying indeed "compared with the novel delights of a society where each moment glittered as it disappeared," and where Mason had "seemed to float upon the broad current of an element theretofore unknown."[28] The difference is that Holmes will give readers of the Breakfast Table books a personal share in these glowing memories, thus permitting them to gaze beyond the narrow bounds of New England culture to a wider horizon:

> do you remember . . . those after-dinners at the Trois Frères, when the Scotch-plaided snuff-box went round, and the dry Lundy-Foot tickled its way along into our happy sensoria? Then it was that the Chambertin or the Clos Vougeot came in, slumbering in its straw cradle. And one among you,—do you remember how he would sit dreaming over his Burgundy, and tinkle his fork against the sides of the bubble-like glass, saying that he was hearing the cow-bells as he used to hear them, when the deep-breathing kine came home at twilight from the huckleberry pasture, in the old home a thousand leagues towards the sunset?[29]

Sunday dinners at the Trois Frères Provençaux, located in the Palais Royale on the Right Bank, were an outgrowth of the daily meetings of the Boston medical students at the Café Procope. The Trois Frères contingent would earn a tiny moment of immortality early in *The Autocrat at the Breakfast Table*, in Holmes's famous peroration on Societies of Mutual Admiration. His own first experience of such a society, he reports, was as the member of a "body of scientific young men in a great foreign city." This was the "Société d'Observation Medicale, of Paris, of which M. Louis was president. . . . They agreed in admiring their justly-honored president, and thought highly of some of their associates."[30] In Boston, readers of Dr. James Jackson, Sr.'s memoir of his son were already familiar with this society. The society was originally very small, the senior Jackson had reported, its active members being "young men, who were proud to call M. Louis their master."[31] Though the Société included medical students from other foreign countries—Holmes's own notification of election was signed by M. Bizot, the Swiss student with whom we earlier saw him cutting up cadavers in the Clamart[32]—its center was the Boston group. The dinners at Trois Frères were simply this same group at their social ease.

In the same way, Holmes interweaves throughout the *Autocrat* memories of Paris that could only belong to a medical student in the 1830s, when he and his Boston friends were following the great hospital teachers on their rounds. So, for instance, a chance association brings into the *Autocrat*'s mind the memory of a little three-year old girl in a French hospital who had fallen out of a chair and broken both thigh bones: "Lying in bed, patient, gentle. Rough students around her, some in white aprons, looking fearfully business-like; but the child placid, perfectly still. I spoke to her, and the blessed little creature answered me in a voice of such heavenly sweetness . . . that I seem to hear it at this moment, while I am writing, so many, many years afterwards.— '*C'est tout comme un serin,*' said the French student at my side."[33] Or the memory, also unbidden, of daily walks homeward through the Latin Quarter—"I used very often," recalls the Autocrat, "when coming home from my morning's work at one of the public institutions of Paris, to stop in at the dear old church of St. Etienne du Mont"[34]—and a medieval Paris to which students from every land had flocked to hear teachers like Albertus Magnus and Aquinas several centuries before any European had set eyes on the coastline of New England.

In place of the revolutionary Paris idolized by democrats like Jefferson and Benjamin Rush, in short—the Paris of Robespierre and the Reign of Terror, of the guillotine and the tumbril, arbitrary arrests and midnight lynchings—*The Autocrat of the Breakfast Table* gradually brings into view another city: the *Paris médicale* of Holmes and his Boston friends, where an open *concours* system decides appointments to the great teaching hospitals, where the French state pays the salaries of the most distinguished physicians and surgeons, where medical students from other countries are not asked to pay for attendance at lectures and clinical teaching, and where no one considers it odd that a dedicated researcher like P. C. A. Louis should devote year after year of unpaid labor to disinterested medical study. The contrast with America could not be more dramatic. If the younger James Jackson were allowed to pursue pure research after returning to the United States, we remember his physician father explaining to Dr. Louis, "he would be regarded as a singular being, governed by a peculiar taste; and it would probably be thought that he would never be fit for the active business of life."[35] In the Paris of the *Autocrat*, no excuse is needed for the pursuit of knowledge—or art, or reading, or even so ordinary an activity as dining—as an end in itself.

As the Trois Frères group had carried Boston with them to Paris—the point, in the passage quoted above, of the "deep-breathing kine" on a remembered New England farm—they bring home with them memories of a Paris where dining in a restaurant, reading a journal in a café, or even greeting an acquaintance on the street belongs to an art of living pursued for its own sake. This is an aspect of Paris existence Holmes had reacted to in the strongest terms during his own days of medical study, as when he wonderingly reports in letters home that linen and table silver are to be found in even the most modest Parisian restaurants, or that like the École de Médecine, the libraries and museums of Paris offer free access to citizens and foreigners alike. Thus, for instance, Holmes's first visit to the Louvre. There were, he reported breathlessly to his parents, nearly one thousand pictures "by the old masters of the Flemish, Dutch, German, and Italian schools. Among them are a large number by Raffael. . . —by Titian—by Rubens—Guido—Salvator Rosa."[36] In the *Autocrat*, an older Holmes will offer the same memories to his readers: "I think Titian understood the look of a gentleman as well as anyone that ever lived. The portrait of a young man holding a glove in his hand, in the Gallery of the Louvre, if any of you have seen that collection, will remind you of what I mean."[37]

The point of such allusions is not to exclude readers who have never been to Europe—if it had been, the *Autocrat* would never have been an overwhelming success with a considerable public—but to situate them in an imaginary world where mention of dinners at the Trois Frères and visits to the Louvre invite them into an atmosphere of cosmopolitan culture. There is such a thing, Holmes will remark in a later volume of the trilogy, "as a lean, impoverished life, as distinct from a rich and suggestive one."[38] He is not talking about Mrs. Trollope's Jacksonian America, the ignorance and crudity of which are by this point simply assumed, but about New England culture as it has not yet transcended its provincial limitations. Throughout the trilogy, it will always be Paris that supplies his standard of genuine civilization. So it is, for instance, that when the Autocrat quotes Thomas Appleton's remark that "Good Americans, when they die, go to Paris," one of the boarders—the school-mistress, to whom the Autocrat will propose marriage at the end of the volume—is compelled to explain to another—the divinity student, who is not yet altogether liberalized in his religious views—that no blasphemy is intended: "It was only another way of saying, Paris is a heavenly place after New York or Boston."[39]

The success of the *Autocrat of the Breakfast Table* was so great that Holmes was easily persuaded to continue the series without a break in *The Professor at the Breakfast Table*, in which the seat of the now-departed Autocrat is taken over by a member of the faculty of a well-known medical school. Along with the change in dramatis personae comes an abrupt alteration of tone. Attentive readers of the first volume had been aware that the Autocrat was someone who had come to view the New England theology of his own childhood as a kind of mental torture imposed on the innocent young—in one of his medical essays Holmes speaks of Bunyan's *Pilgrim's Progress*, put into the hands of New England children as a matter of course, as filled with "nightmare dreams of horror"[40]—and that this conclusion has something to do with his medical studies in Paris. In *The Professor*, the veil is lifted. The speaker at the breakfast table is now a Paris-trained physician wholly conversant with modern discoveries in physics, biology, chemistry, and geology, to whom his scientific studies have suggested a set of metaphysical assumptions that leave him no choice but to speak as an inveterate foe of Calvin's nightmare doctrines of predestination and Total Depravity.

The importance of the Professor's Paris experience is that, at a crucial moment in his intellectual development, it had given him an outside perspective on New England religious culture. "I left the paternal roof," he will tell his readers at one point, "and wandered in other lands, and learned to think in the words of a strange people."[41] As he appears in this Breakfast Table volume, he is already an experienced controversialist, known to the public as an implacable opponent of pseudo-science and quackery, and in medical circles as the victor in a bitter disagreement among physicians over the contagiousness of puerperal fever. The Professor is thus ready to agree with a fellow boarder, as fearless in controversy as himself, that "A man whose opinions are not attacked is beneath contempt." "I hope so," responds the Professor, for when, several years before, he had "held up to the professional public the damnable facts connected with the conveyance of poison from one young mother's chamber to another's,—for doing which humble office I desire to be thankful that I have lived, though nothing else good should ever come of my life,—I had to bear the sneers of those whose position I had assailed, and, as I believe, have at last demolished, so that nothing but the ghosts of dead women stir among the ruins."[42]

The controversy on which *The Professor of the Breakfast Table* now embarks concerns the variety of Calvinism called New England theology, whose brilliant and chilling expositor had been the famous Jonathan Edwards of Northampton, Massachusetts. For Edwards had taught with great power and eloquence that predestination was the sole doctrine compatible with God's omniscience—to say that God was ignorant of anything whatever, including whether or not any soul born into the world would be damned or saved, would be impermissibly to subtract from His divinity —and that the doctrine of Total Depravity, making every human being worthy of damnation due to Adam and Eve's sin, was more than enough to explain why will or volition can play no role in the economy of eternal salvation. In Edwards's stern Calvinism, men are thus born hateful to God—a human being is, in the usual language of New England theology, "a little, wretched, despicable creature; a worm, a mere nothing and less than nothing"[43]—and only a tiny number are to be saved through God's mercy. The rest, an overwhelming majority, are born predestined to an eternity of torment. This is the theology that persisted, in Holmes's view, as a lingering blight on New England thought.

In Edwards's sermons, Holmes surmised, the preacher who so obsessively dwelt on the horrors of hell as a divine torture-chamber had given clear evidence of a disordered imagination. But even this was less pathological than his position on infant damnation. The doctrine of Original Sin has always found itself in a hard place with respect to the newborn child, who is on the one hand damned because the inheritor of Adam's guilt, but on the other seemingly innocent because incapable of willing any action at all. Yet no one who believes in Original Sin, Edwards had argued, will attempt to deny that such infants "are *justly* treated as sinners, truly guilty, and *children of wrath.*"[44] So it is, Holmes remarks with elaborate irony, that the little "automaton is not sent into the world without an inheritance. Every infant . . . is entitled to one undivided share of the guilt and consequent responsibility of the Trustee to whom the Sovereign had committed its future."[45] Nor are the natural affections of a parent any argument against this fate. On Edwards's view, parents who are among God's elect "will sing hallelujahs as they see their children driven into the flames."[46]There are, remarks Holmes drily, "conceptions which are not only false, not only absurd, but which act as *disorganizing forces* in the midst of the thinking apparatus."

Holmes's focus on Edwards is so unremitting, in both the Breakfast Table series and other writings, that it could easily enough be mistaken for a personal animus. Thus, for instance, in an essay on Edwards published in 1880, he describes with a kind of fascinated horror the effects of Edwards's preaching on the people of his Northampton parish: "Faintings, convulsions, utter prostration, trances, visions like those of delirium tremens, were common occurrences. Children went home from the religious meetings crying aloud through the streets. Some lost their reason; . . . While the work was at its height a poor man, overwhelmed with melancholy, made an attempt to cut his throat. Then a gentleman of good standing, who had been greatly concerned about the state of his soul, but who 'durst entertain no hope concerning his own good estate,' succeeded in taking his life in that way."[47] Yet the essence of Holmes's analysis is that Calvinism was itself, long before Edwards came on the scene, already a deranged theology. In his personal notebook, Holmes would transcribe from Hippolyte Taine a passage—the subject is the poet William Cowper's attempts at suicide—describing "the profound dejection, gloomy and continual despair, the horrible malady of the nerves and the soul which leads to suicide, Puritanism, and madness."[48]

At the heart of the Professor's warfare against New Engand theology lies a more general conviction that prescriptive religious doctrines, from the Total Depravity of Calvinism to Roman Catholic transubstantiation to the Thirty-Nine Articles of Anglicanism, can in the nature of things be no more than examples of human presumption, attempts to contain the mystery of an infinite universe within the narrow limits of a merely human creed. His own experience in medical controversy gave Holmes some warrant for thinking that all that was needed to expose such presumption was freedom of discussion. Yet here the stakes were higher, for Boston, as Holmes well knew, had means, ranging from social disapproval to outright ostracism, to punish members of its community who dared to raise their voices against Calvinist orthodoxy. In *The Professor at the Breakfast Table,* the representative of this orthodoxy is the divinity student, who is recurrently scandalized by the Professor's outspokenness. "You would not," he asks reproachfully, "attack a church dogma—say Total Depravity—in a lyceum lecture, for instance." The Professor quite agrees: a lecturer is an invited guest, and is bound to honor the taboos and prejudices of his audience. But, he adds, "at this table I think it is very different. I shall express my ideas on any subject I like."[49]

In *The Professor,* Holmes's imaginary breakfast table gradually becomes a magical space in which opinions never before publicly heard in Boston are not only fearlessly uttered, but meant to be overheard by a large audience of *Atlantic Monthly* readers throughout the English-speaking world. "I shall not often give arguments," the Professor tells the divinity student, "but frequently opinions,—I trust with courtesy and propriety, but, at any rate, with such natural forms of expression as it has pleased the Almighty to bestow upon me."[50] The mention of the Almighty gives us, in conventional religious language, the essential relation between

Holmes's own metaphysics of consciousness and his insistence on liberty of discussion: in a world otherwise governed by deterministic physical laws, the rational intellect alone is free. To restrict its activity would be, in a manner of speaking, the highest imaginable blasphemy against rational consciousness. Many of Holmes's readers, including his friend James Russell Lowell, found the new tone exhilarating. "I like the new Professor," wrote Lowell shortly after the appearance of the first number, "better than the old Autocrat." " The Religious Press . . . will be at you, but after smashing one of them you will be able to furnish yourself with a Sampson's weapon for the rest of the Philistines."[51]

The religious press had, in fact, been attacking Holmes for years. In *The Professor at the Breakfast Table* it would become clear, however, that his real object all along had less to do with theology than with a deeper transformation of Boston intellectual culture. In succeeding numbers, the Calvinist doctrines to which the divinity student still adheres give way to the radical demand for free inquiry voiced by the character whom the boarders call Little Boston, whose physical deformation—shrunken body, twisted limbs, limping gait—mirrors the spiritual deformation wrought upon the New England mind by Puritan writers like Cotton Mather and preachers like Jonathan Edwards. Little Boston, the last surviving member of an old Massachusetts family, is the grandson of an innocent woman hanged as a witch in the Salem trials. Yet his fierce pride in Boston remains undiminished, to the point that his praise of his native city is really a mode of moral exhortation, reminding his listeners that Massachusetts, alone among the American colonies, had been founded in the name of spiritual liberty: "A new race, and a whole new world for the new-born human soul to work in! And Boston is the brain of it, and has been any time these hundred years. That's all I claim for Boston,—that it is the thinking centre of the continent, and therefore of the planet."[52]

Most readers of the *Atlantic* understood immediately that Little Boston—or, as he comes to be known as the boarders grow fond of him, the Little Gentleman—was Holmes's self-parody of his own well-known local attachment to Boston. Yet beneath the parody lies a serious point. The Puritans who founded the Massachusetts colony had made a heroic break with the prescriptive religious doctrines of an older European world: with Roman Catholicism, to be sure, in the Reformation of Luther and Calvin, but then also with the seventeenth-century Anglican church whose Thirty-Nine articles and ecclesiastical structure had driven a tiny group of English Puritans to the wilderness of an unexplored New World. This is the sense in which the rigid orthodoxy of later New England theology might be legitimately viewed as a betrayal of the Puritan ideal of religious freedom, as well as of its offshoot in the spirit of political freedom that had made Bostonians like Samuel Adams and James Otis prime movers of the America Revolution. In demanding that nineteenth-century Boston culture return to its own intellectual origins, Little Boston thus becomes the voice of what Holmes elsewhere calls spiritual republicanism:

> A man can see further, Sir,—he said one day,—from the top of the Boston State House, and see more that is worth seeing, than from all the pyramids and turrets and steeples in all the places of the world! No smoke, Sir; no fog, Sir; and a clean sweep from the Outer Light and the sea beyond it to the New Hampshire mountains! Yes, Sir,—and there are great truths that are higher than mountains and broader than seas, that people are looking for from the tops of these hills of ours,—such as the world never saw, though it might have seen them at Jersusalem, if its eyes had been open![53]

The ground of free discussion cleared by Little Boston's repeated exhortations is then occupied by the Professor in, specifically, his role as a physician and teacher of medicine. In the course of *The Professor at the Breakfast Table* we encounter many of the instances of medical fraud and error discussed in Holmes's medical essays, but now his point will always be that prescriptive religion is to the soul what medical quackery is to the body. Both play to human credulity and selfishness, holding out perpetual health or the soul's immortality as the prize for taking just this or that remedy or believing this or that theological doctrine. Nor will the world ever lack for mountebanks, spiritual or physical, to exploit human weakness. "A few score years ago," the Professor recalls, "sick people were made to swallow burnt toads and powdered earthworms. . . . The physician of Charles I and II prescribed abominations not to be named. Traces of this barbarism linger even in the greatly improved medical science of our century. So while the solemn farce of over-drugging is going on, the world over, the harlequin pseudo-science jumps on to the stage, whip in hand, with half-a-dozen somersets, and begins laying about him."[54]

At the same time, there are in religion, as in medicine, varieties of quackery—that improbable folly of the world, as the Professor calls it, that so often confounds wisdom[55]— that in a theological perspective would be seen as providential. So, in medicine, it took the pseudo-science of homeopathy, with its infinitesimal doses, to dupe patients into thinking they were being treated even as they were unwittingly escaping the terrible consequences of the bleeding, drugging, purging system that had undermined the health of their parents and grandparents. In theology, says the Professor, much the same purpose is now being served by Spiritualism, with its promises of putting the living into communication with the souls of the departed. For when one looks past the obvious fraudulence of such claims, what remains is an altered conception of the immortality of the soul: instead of Jonathan Edwards's fiery torture-chamber of eternal damnation, one now imagines something very like a democracy of ghosts.[56] "Spiritualism," the Professor observes, "is quietly undermining the traditional ideas of the future state which have been and are still accepted,—not merely in those who believe in it, but in the general sentiment of the community. . . . It needn't be true, to do this, any more than Homœpathy need, to do its work."[57]

The point of the analogy between medical and religious quackery is that they are based on an identical logic: once a mistaken premise is established, virtually any system may be made internally consistent with itself. So, for instance, a physician who accepts the premises of humoral theory—the four bodily fluids corresponding to the four elements of earth, air, fire, and water—is being perfectly reasonable to bleed the patient for plethora. The homeopathist, operating on an erroneous analogy between his own infinitesimal doses and vaccination for smallpox, is quite right to give a sick person a grain of quinine diluted to the billionth part. In *The Professor at the Breakfast Table*, the most sustained analogy is with the relatively new science of Phrenology. If one accepts the premise that the organs of the brain determine human character, and if the relative development of those organs in an individual may be estimated by bumps in the formation of the skull, then phrenological analysis is both rigorous and reasonable. Exactly how, though, would one go about proving that such a premise is erroneous? The Professor's reductio ad absurdum returns us to the guiding principles of Paris medicine:

> The walls of the head are double, with a great air-chamber between them, over the smallest and most closely crowded "organs." Can you tell how much money there is in a safe, which also has thick double walls, by kneading its knobs with your fingers? So when a man fumbles about my forehead, and talks about the organs of *Individuality, Size*, etc., I trust him as much as I should if he felt of the outside of my strong-box and told me that there was a five-dollar or a ten-dollar-bill under this or that particular rivet. Perhaps there is; *only he doesn't know anything about it.*[58]

Holmes's treatment of theological doctrine is similar. If one grants Calvin his conception of God's omniscience, the principle of predestination follows with perfect consistency. In the same way, if one accepts the Bible as a source of scientific evidence, the inferences that permitted Bishop Ussher to set the date of the Creation at 4004 B.C. are logical and coherent. This is a notion Holmes has fun with in *The Poet at the Breakfast Table* when the Poet, tiptoeing through what he knows to be a theological minefield, hesitantly asks the learned polymath called the Master what he thinks of Darwinian theory. The Master's reply is a sly exercise in peremptory irony: "Better stick to Blair's Chronology; that settles it. Adam and Eve, created Friday, October 28, B.C. 4004."[59] But, as in the case of phrenology, a mistaken premise can only lead to solemn nonsense: Bishop Ussher was not a geologist, and had no business computing the age of the earth. The error of phrenology, similarly, is that it is ignorant about cerebral anatomy, which is why Holmes, as a teacher of anatomy, allows himself a rare moment of dogmatism in pronouncing on it: "this is a point that I, the Professor, understand, my friends, or ought to, certainly, better than you do."[60]

The superiority of scientific truth is thus that it does not begin from a priori dogmatisms, but from such demonstrable evidence as the space between the cerebrum and the bones of the skull, or the presence of marine fossils in the geologic strata of hills and mountains. Yet the Breakfast Table trilogy dwells on the paradox that such facts as these lead more surely than religious dogma to a sense of genuine mystery, just as the vast stretches of geologic time opened up by Lyell or Darwin move the imagination more surely towards the sense of an infinite cosmos than Bishop Ussher's creation date of 4000 B.C. In nearby Roxbury and Dorchester, the Professor once muses, boys are fond of breaking off pieces of what they call puddingstone, without ever understanding that it once lay at the bottom of a prehistoric sea: "Yet a lump of puddingstone is a thing to look at, to think about, to study over, to dream upon. . . . Look at that pebble in it. From what cliff was it broken? On what beach rolled by the waves of what ocean? How and *when* imbedded in soft ooze, which itself became stone, and by-and-by was lifted into bald summits and steep cliffs, such as you may see on Meetinghouse-Hill any day?"[61]

The paradox occurs because there is no mystery in facts as such. The sense of mystery can only arise—this is the point of Holmes's talk about thinking, studying, dreaming—within human consciousness. It is at such moments that Holmes goes beyond Paley's *Natural Theology*. Paley had imagined that the order discovered in nature must imply intelligent design, and that the more complex nature turned out to be—as in, especially, the wondrous complexity of living organisms—the more powerful would be the demonstration of a divine intent. Holmes, on the other hand, had seen very clearly that something like Darwin's theory might well arrive to explain even the most complex organism as a product of blind natural processes, the laws of physics and chemistry in their ceaseless and eternal operations. This is why Holmes will always go out of his way to emphasize that the real mystery concerns the mind that postulates or grasps physical laws: "It is a mistake . . . to think the mystery is greater in an organized body than in any other. We see a stone fall or a crystal form, and there is nothing stranger left to wonder at, for we have seen the Infinite in action. . . . If the sovereign Artificer lets us into his own laboratories and workshops, we need not ask more than the privilege of looking on at his work."[62]

The Professor at the Breakfast Table marks the moment when Holmes takes on the role of spiritual physician to an age deeply troubled by religious doubt. "We are all theological students," he had said in the *Autocrat*, "and more of us qualified as doctors of divinity than have received degrees."[63] By the time the series was in its second volume, it was clear to many readers that the Breakfast Table books were underwritten by a clear and consistent set of metaphysical assumptions. "It would be interesting," said Holmes's contemporary biographer W. S. Kennedy, "to draw up a *Religio Medici*, extracting from his books the doctrines which he believes as well as those he has combated in so many places and on so many occasions."[64] Kennedy's reference is to the *Religio Medici*—'a physician's religion'—of Sir Thomas Browne, the great seventeenth-century author of *Hydriotaphia* and other meditational writings, who along with Samuel Johnson counts as one of the primary influences on Holmes's thought and writing. In *The Professor* and *The Poet*, especially, the Norwich physician is summoned again and again as a witness in favor of Holmes's own metaphysics of consciousness.

In one sense, the influence of *Religio Medici* on Holmes's thought and writing seems simple enough to explain. For Browne, like Holmes, had been a physician trained in Europe at a time when science was radically altering conceptions of the physical universe and the human body, as in Galileo's elaboration of Copernican theory or Harvey's discovery of the circulation, which Browne once said he preferred to the discoveries of Columbus.[65] But what most drew Holmes to *Religio Medici*, it seems clear, had to do with a certain timeless element in the physician's relation to the world, one that would have been as immediately intelligible to Hippocrates or Galen as to any graduate of a nineteenth-century medical school. In any age of civilization, it is the physician who works on a daily basis at the mysterious intersection of body and soul. "In our study of anatomy," Browne says in *Religio Medici*, "there is a mass of mysterious philosophy."[66] Consider the Professor's report, for the benefit of the other boarders at the breakfast table, on the most recent news concerning the structure and function of hemoglobin:

How many "swimming glands"—solid, organized, regularly formed, rounded disks taking an active part in all your vital processes, part and parcel, each one of them, of your corporeal being—do you suppose are whirled along, like pebbles in a stream, with the blood which warms your frame. . . ? A noted German physiologist spread out a minute drop of blood, under the microscope, in narrow streaks, and counted the globules, and then made a calculation. The counting by the micrometer took him *a week.*—You have, my full-grown friend, of these little couriers in crimson or scarlet livery, running on your vital errands day and night as long as you live, sixty-five billions, five hundred and seventy thousand millions.[67]

To read such passages against the background of Paley's *Natural Theology*, as many *Atlantic* readers no doubt did, is to find oneself on the familiar ground of miraculous design. Nor is this entirely nonsensical. Even today, the complex system through which hemoglobin transports oxygen, or the molecular structure that gives the erythrocyte its extraordinary oxygen-carrying capacity, can provoke an unbidden sense of wonder in the beginning student. But that is not the Professor's point. It is that *science* is the miracle: the notion of the body as a self-contained physiological system pioneered by the great French anatomists, the compound microscope, only recently developed due to an improved understanding of the laws of refraction, Virchow's isolation of the cell as the basic unit of life, all combining to create the human body as a marvelous mental construct intelligible as such only to beings endowed with rational consciousness. "We do not know where we now stand in the hierarchy of created intelligences," says Holmes in one of his medical essays. "We were *made* a little lower than the angels. I speak it not irreverently; as the lower animals surpass man in some of their attributes, so it may be that not every angel's eye can see as broadly and as deeply into the material works of God as man himself, looking at the firmament through an equatorial of fifteen inches aperture, and searching into the tissues with a twelfth of an inch objective."[68]

At any such moment, Holmes's metaphysics of consciousness in the Breakfast Table trilogy moves very close to the central principle of Browne's *Religio Medici*, which is that in a blind physical universe—what Holmes himself once calls "the world of unconscious matter"[69]— the world would in an important sense be as though it had never come into existence. Browne's way of putting the matter uses the Biblical vocabulary of an earlier age, but the point, as Holmes would have maintained, is just as compelling in the new world of cell biology and compound microscopes as it had been in the days of Harvey and the Royal Society. "The world," says Browne, "was made to be . . . studied and contemplated by man; 'tis the debt of our reason we owe unto God." For in the absence of human consciousness, the universe would still be "as though it had not been, or as it was before the sixth day when as yet there was not a creature that could conceive or say there was a world."[70] In *The Poet at the Breakfast Table*, the Poet will give his own version of the same point in discussion with the young Astronomer: "conscious life is the grand aim and end of all this vast mechanism. Without life that could feel and enjoy, the splendors and creative energy would all be thrown away."[71]

Still, the simple intuition of the primacy of consciousness is as old as religion and philosophy. To philosophers like Plato and Plotinus, it seemed self-evident that rational consciousness, moving freely as it does in an immaterial world of mathematical and artistic and moral truth, could not belong to the realm of brute matter. In theological terms, the same point is made by Milton's Belial when, in *Paradise Lost*, he argues that even amidst the torments of Hell the existence of the fallen angels is preferable to their annihilation as conscious beings: "for who would lose, Though full of pain, this intellectual being, Those thoughts that wander through eternity, To perish rather, swallowed up and lost In the wide womb of uncreated night, Devoid of sense and motion?"[72] In Augustine, taking over from Plotinus the notion that the soul in this world is in a state of exile from a higher realm of pure spirit, the same intuition proves the truth of the Judeo-Christian theological tradition, from the creation of Adam and Eve to the Resurrection. For the Augustine of the *Confessions*, visited in the moment of his conversion by a vision of mortal life as a tragic state of alienation from God, what was yesterday merely a myth has today become a divinely-inspired narrative with enormous explanatory power.

In religio-philosophical terms, one clear implication of the metaphysics of consciousness is that the body is, so to speak, disposable. This is Socrates' point in arguing that the soul is truest to its own nature when it flees the body, and the point of Plotinus in describing imprisonment in the physical body as a state of exile from the One. In the religio medici of both Browne and Holmes—I dispense with italics from now on—a version of the same point, familiar to physicians throughout the ages, is that the soul inhabits many bodies throughout its mortal span. This is what Browne has in mind, for instance, in observing that *All flesh is grass* is literally true, "for all those creatures we behold, are but the herbs of the field, digested into flesh in them, or more remotely carnified in ourselves." "All this mass of flesh which we behold," he adds—and here he means our own bodies—"came in at our mouths; this frame we look upon, hath been upon our trenchers."[73] The same theme recurs constantly in Holmes's writing. The persistence of consciousness independent of any particular body is simply a fact of nature. For the existence of living beings is "a perpetual death and reanimation. Their identity is only an idea, for we put off our bodies many times during our lives, and dress in new suits of bones and muscles."[74]

Yet the physician, whose very vocation demands that he treat the body as a physical system, deals daily with the alternative possibility that consciousness may be a mere epiphenomenon of matter in its endless combinations. This thought, too, is very old, going back to the atomism of Democritus in Greek philosophy and works like Lucretius' *De Rerum Naturae* in the Roman world. It is a thought that is never very far from Holmes's mind, especially in the form of the Scholastic phrase—*Ubi tres medici, duo athei:* 'where there are three physicians, you will find two atheists'[75]—to which he recurs again and again in his writings. In Browne's *Religio Medici*, it arises in the lines from Seneca's *Troades* that would haunt the European mind from the time of Bacon's *Novum Organon* on: *Post mortem nihil est, ipsaque mors nihil,* . . . *Tempus nos avidum devorat et chaos*—'After death there is nothing, and death itself is nothing . . . Remorseless time and chaos wait to devour us.' Or, in the splendid version by Browne's contemporary the Earl of Rochester, "Dead, we become the lumber of the world,   And to that mass of matter shall be swept Where things destroyed with things unborn are kept."[76] This is precisely the dark vision that would come back to haunt Victorian religion in the age of Lyell and Darwin.

At the same time, the physician is daily witness to a power in the universe that works towards regeneration, healing, and a continual reprieve, during the span granted to any living individual, from death and decay. This is the *vis medicatrix naturae*, whose central role in Browne's *Religio Medici*, as in Holmes's medical essays, derives directly from his own perspective as a healer of the sick. Most people, who are healthy most of the time, take health as something like a natural right, illness as a personal insult or an interruption in the order of nature. But the physician, living in a world of disease and death, sees things otherwise. "Men that look no further than their outsides think health an appurtenance unto life," says Browne somewhat wryly, "and quarrel with their constitutions for being sick; but I have that have examined the parts of man, and know upon what tender filaments that fabric hangs, do wonder that we are not always so; and considering the thousand doors that lead to death do thank my God that we can die but once."[77] It is the same thought that Holmes has in mind whenever he points out, speaking as a physician, that to tend the sick is to spend one's life in the perpetual presence of the "great Healing Agent, who stays the bleeding of wounds" and "who knits the fractured bone."[78]

In Holmes's writings, the *vis medicatrix* lies at the center of the system of metaphysical assumptions he opposes both to the Calvinist orthodoxy of his New England boyhood and to the modern philosophical materialism that, having achieved intellectual respectability in Enlightenment France, has now entered the mainstream of nineteenth-century thought. From the perspective of the *vis medicatrix* there is a certain resemblance between the Hell of Jonathan Edwards—that torture chamber where damned souls spend their sleepless eternity—and the universe as a blind whirl of matter— the *tempus avidum et chaos* of Seneca's lines—that remains perpetually oblivious to the fact of human existence. In opposing the *vis medicatrix* to religious notions of Hell or damnation, Holmes will ordinarily stress the sense in which it argues a solicitude for the fate of living creatures: "It is impossible, or at least very difficult, for a physician who has seen the perpetual efforts of Nature—whose diary is the book he reads oftenest—to heal wounds, to expel poisons . . . —it is very difficult for him to believe in a world where wounds cannot heal, where opiates cannot give a respite from pain, . . . where the art of torture is the only science cultivated, and the capacity for being tormented is the only faculty which remains to the children of that same Father who cares for the falling sparrow."[79]

In dealing with the dead universe of modern scientific materialism, on the other hand, Holmes will normally stress the power of consciousness to grasp the *vis medicatrix* as a metaphysical principle—or, by extension, to postulate the very physical laws through which science explains electromagnetism or cell biology—as setting a limit to what can be explained by physics or chemistry. "Mr. Huxley maintains," Holmes once wryly remarks, "that his thoughts and ours are 'the expression of molecular changes in that matter of life which is the source of our other vital phenomena'."[80] Holmes's implicit point will always be that such materialist dogmatism sounds suspiciously like the dogmatism of theologians like Calvin or medical faddists like Hahnemann, in which a single large premise, asserted rather than proved, is made to serve as the foundation of an elaborate system. He leaves it to the Professor, as a scientifically-trained physician, to express the sense of mystery that seems to him inseparable from his own existence as a conscious being:

> I have many times stopped short and held my breath, and felt the blood leaving my cheeks, in one of these sudden clairvoyant flashes. Of course I cannot tell what kind of a secret this is, but I think of it as a disclosure of certain relations of our personal being to time and space, to other intelligences, and to their First Great Cause. This secret seems to be broken up, as it were, into fragments, so that we find here a word and there a syllable, and then again only a letter of it; but it never is written out for most of us as a complete sentence, in this life.[81]

The Poet at the Breakfast Table, with which Holmes was prevailed upon to bring the series to a conclusion in 1870, is largely an exposition of that metaphysics of consciousness with which *The Professor* had been so largely occupied. Even as early as *The Autocrat*, which had begun by projecting a miscellaneous audience, Holmes had toward the end begun to assume the voice of a preacher addressing a religious congregation.

"Our parish is so large," he says at one point, explaining why his conversation so often mixes humor and serious discussion, "one can't pretend to preach to all the pews at once."[82] By the time he reaches *The Poet*, this audience has been reduced to a single universalized reader, always addressed as "Beloved," in which readers were meant to recognize an echo of the "dearly beloved" or "dearly beloved of the Lord" of the *Book of Common Prayer.* Nor were readers unaware that in this last volume religious or theological preoccupations had moved to the center of the Breakfast Table discourse. The hopes of Abiel Holmes that his son would feel a calling to the ministry were not, observed W.S. Kennedy, altogether absurd: "There is a good deal of the preacher in Holmes; his essays are lay sermons."[83]

In *The Poet*, the boarding house has changed as well. From the representative social types of the *Autocrat*, deliberately imitating the random social mix of Mrs. Trollope's *Domestic Manners of the Americans*, the breakfast table company has gradually become an intellectual community, a microcosm of Boston culture as Holmes himself saw it epitomized in the Saturday Club or the monthly *Atlantic* dinners.[84] "I think we have a somewhat exceptional company," says the Poet at the beginning of the new series, explaining that the Landlady, ever since an earlier boarder of hers brought her establishment into notice—he means, of course, the Autocrat—"has been decidedly a favorite with persons a little above the average in point of intelligence and education." One consequence has been that the company now seated around the breakfast table includes "a considerable number of literary and scientific people." Another is that "there is more individuality of character than in a good many similar boarding houses, where"—it is the last glance Holmes's series will take at the boarding houses of Mrs. Trollope's Jacksonian America—"all are business-minded, engrossed in the same pursuit of money-getting, or all are engaged in politics."[85]

The three major spokesmen for Holmes's metaphysics of consciousness at this breakfast table are the Poet of the title, the Master, a learned polymath conversant with the latest discoveries of experimental science, and the Astronomer, a young man from a well-to-do family who has chosen to devote himself to the study of the cosmos, spending his nights in a cold observatory making detailed observations of the planets, stars, and remotest galaxies. It is the Master, a student of the classics and an author as well as a scientist, who sees that the young Astronomer's scientific studies are also a kind of poetry. "You call yourself a Poet," he says to his fellow boarder. "But that young man lives in a world beyond the imagination of poets, let me tell you. The daily home of his thought is in illimitable space, hovering between the two eternities."[86] And the Poet, when he has come to know the young man, agrees: "He seems more like one who has come from a planet farther away from the sun than our earth. . . . A strange unearthly being; lonely, dwelling far apart from the thoughts and cares of the planet on which he lives,—an enthusiast who gives his life to knowledge; a student of antiquity, to whom the records of the geologist are modern pages in the great volume of being, and the pyramids a memorandum of yesterday."[87]

The province of the Poet in this final volume is, on the other hand, the dimension of rational consciousness that permits human societies to dwell within shared structures of transcendent possibility. This is the moral sense theory that, originating with Shaftesbury in the eighteenth century, would have so important an influence on such philosophers as Rousseau and Kant. For Holmes, its significance would always be that the moral sense—for him, as for Shaftesbury and Kant, nearly allied with the aesthetic—marks the radical division between mere sentience and rational consciousness. Sentience is a property of the animal creation from the earthworm to the kangaroo, but only to human intelligence is it given to perceive virtue in actions—meaning, as well as right conduct, such qualities as courage and fortitude and honesty and generosity of spirit—or beauty in art and nature. Holmes's usual name for the moral sense, given currency by Adam Smith's *Theory of Moral Sentiments*, was "sentiment":

> It does not go a great way in deciding questions of arithmetic, or alge-
> bra, or geometry. . . . But inasmuch as religion and law and the whole
> social order of civilized society, to say nothing of literature and art, are so
> founded on and pervaded by sentiment that they would all go to pieces
> without it, it is a word not to be used too lightly in passing judgment, as if
> it were an element to be thrown out or treated with small consideration.
> Reason may be the lever, but sentiment gives you the fulcrum and the
> place to stand on if you want to move the world.[88]

Yet the final spokesman for Holmes's religio medici is the Master—his name recalling the *Magister Artium* of medieval scholasticism—whose Pasteur-like microbial experiments recall Holmes's own medical train- ing and teaching, whose love of Greek and Latin literature is at one with Holmes's lifelong devotion to humanistic learning, and whose view of modern science is, like that of Holmes, shot through with a sense of infinite mystery, as with the singularly perfect and beautiful specimen of a fossil trilobite the Master keeps by him when writing at his desk: "Look here!—he said. I keep oblivion always before me. . . . Each time I fill a sheet of paper with what I am writing, I lay it beneath this relic of a dead world. . . . Our world, too, with all its breathing life, is but a leaf to be folded with the other strata, and if I am only patient, by and by I shall be just as famous as imperious Caesar himself, embedded with me in a conglomerate."[89] In the echo of Hamlet's graveyard speech, itself an echo of the medieval *memento mori* tradition, lies Holmes's reminder to readers in the age of Lyell and Darwin that human consciousness has never, even when in the act of imagining its own extinction, been wholly able to rid itself of intimations of its own immortality.

In the Master's concluding ruminations on his own writings we hear as well Holmes's thoughts on his career as author of the Breakfast Table series, so unexpectedly gotten under way in the pages of the *Atlantic* nearly a quarter century after his return from Paris, but drawing constantly on those alterations in his own thinking that had begun in the wards of La Pitié and at the dissecting tables of the Clamart: "*Liveravi animam meam.* That is the meaning of my book and of my literary life, if I may give such a name to that parti-colored shred of human existence. I have unburdened myself in this book, and in some other pages, of what I was born to say. . . . I do know this: I have struck a good many chords, first and last, in the consciousness of other people" And, a little later: "I have got rid of something my mind could not keep to itself and rise as it was meant to into higher regions."[90] As the thousands of letters he received from readers would demonstrate, it was not simply his own mind that Holmes permitted to rise into higher regions. "No philosophy or theory of life will be known by his name," wrote William Dean Howells after Holmes's death. ". . . He was essentially observant, and in this he showed the scientific nature." But his works accomplished what can only be done by the great moralists: Holmes brought his readers, says Howells, to an understanding of themselves, "first in the little, and then in the larger things."[91]

For a great number of readers throughout the English-speaking world, Holmes's Breakfast Table books, continuously drawing on an inexhaustible fertility of imagination, were themselves a dramatization of the very metaphysics of consciousness on which his own religio medici was based. As such, the books would have a profound influence on their own time. Holmes lived on into the last decade of the nineteenth century. There is something very nearly elegiac in the series of prefaces he would supply to successive editions of his Breakfast Table volumes, increasingly going forth as the years went by into a world that they themselves had done a great deal to create. The trouble with offering books like *The Professor at the Breakfast Table* to readers today, Holmes observes in a preface written in 1880, is "that their heresies have become so familiar among intelligent people that they have too commonplace an aspect." Still, though "all the lighthouses and land-marks of belief" have altered remarkably in the interim, it is essential to realize that modern spiritual anxiety is, after all, part of an age-old human story, and that, as Holmes says reassuringly to a new generation of readers now looking tremulously toward a modernity that may turn out to be even more troubling to the spirit, "we and our fellow-passengers are still in the same old vessel sailing the same unfathomable sea and bound to the same as yet unseen harbor."[92]

Note on Sources

The scholarly literature on the Paris clinical revolution is extensive and of very high quality. One of the great pleasures of working on this book, if I may be permitted to say so, has been to find myself in a field where scholars are still moved by a genuine sense of vocation. During the happy hours I spent buried in past issues of the *Bulletin of the History of Medicine* and such splendid scholarly works as Jacalyn Duffin's biography of R. T. H. Laennec and Othmar Keel's *La généalogie de l'histopathologie,* I was reminded many times of the enlivening sense of common intellectual purpose that existed when I began in literary studies nearly forty years ago. Younger scholars in history of medicine are fortunate indeed to have entered their field in that dawn when it is, as Wordsworth said about his own era, a bliss to be alive.

The seminal work that stands behind all current scholarship on Paris medicine is Ackerknecht's *Medicine at the Paris Hospital.* Ackerknecht produced, as well, a number of classic essays that do not duplicate material in that study. It is the highest of compliments to his work that contemporary studies in Paris medicine still tend to be either elaborations of Ackerknecht, modifications of Ackerknecht, or refutations of Ackerknecht. For those not in history of medicine, the one problem with *Medicine at the Paris Hospital* is that it assumes a good deal of prior knowledge of its field: when the names of Chomel or Andral or Alibert or Amussat mean something to a reader, Ackerknecht's dense work seems luminous in its ability to lay bare connections and isolate affiliations. When the same names mean nothing at all, his presentation can sometimes seem like a congested list of names and dates. One of my hopes in writing *Oliver Wendell Holmes in Paris* has been, in fact, that readers with no prior knowledge of history of medicine might end the book feeling enough at home in what Ackerknecht called the Paris hospital to go on to read both his work and others mentioned in this note.

Medicine at the Paris Hospital was published in 1967. Just over thirty years later, a second important introductory work appeared—"introductory" not in the sense that it simplifies its presentation for beginners, but that it permits outsiders to the field to navigate its scholarly domain without losing their bearings. The work is *Constructing Paris Medicine*, edited by Caroline Hannaway and Ann La Berge. The mariner's compass they provide is their own splendidly comprehensive and lucid introductory chapter: "Paris Medicine: Perspectives Past and Present." *Constructing Paris Medicine* appeared when I had already been at work on Holmes's medical studies for most of a decade. I wish that it had been there at the beginning of my research.

Readers of my notes will see how indebted I have been both to Hannaway and La Berge and to certain of their contributors—especially L. W. B. Brockliss, Othmar Keel, and W. R. Albury. A bonus for readers interested in this important chapter in modern medical history is the bibliography to the volume, which includes a good deal of important archival material as well as an indispensable list of secondary sources. My own present note on sources would have been a great deal longer if *Constructing Paris Medicine* had not appeared just when it did. As it is, I will simply content myself with referring readers to Hannaway and La Berge's excellent bibliography.

One item in that bibliography deserves separate mention. This is Jacalyn Duffin's *To See With a Better Eye*, a monumental and exciting biography of R. T. H. Laennec that in itself changes the way scholars specializing in Paris medicine view, especially, the period between Bichat's *Anatomie générale* and Laennec's *De l'auscultation médiate*. Only a long period in the bewildering labyrinth of the Laennec archives, plus a great deal of scholarly insight and ingenuity, could have produced so magisterial a work. One suspects that its feel for clinical or bedside medicine was aided, in addition, by Dr. Duffin's being an M.D. as well as a distinguished historian of French medicine. In her subsequent *History of Medicine*, a short introductory work written specifically for medical students, her presentation of Laennec's discovery as a *coupure épistémologique*—what in my first chapter I call the "discovery of disease," or the new concept of disease as an autonomous entity—is attractively situated in a longer-term historical perspective. As a bonus for those interested in doing further work in the field, Duffin's *History of Medicine* contains an invaluable section—Appendix B: "Resources and Research Tools for the History of Medicine"—providing guidance to beginning scholars, or scholars in other areas who find their work intersecting the history of medicine at some vital point.

On the American side of the Atlantic, two works had an enormous impact on my own thinking about Holmes and Paris medicine. The first is Russell M. Jones's *The Parisian Education of An American Surgeon*, an edition of Jonathan Mason Warren's letters to his father in the years 1832–1835, plus the series of specialized articles on American doctors in Paris written by Jones during the same period he was editing those letters. My own interest in Holmes and Paris medicine goes back to the time when I first read this book some twenty-five years ago. The other major work for those interested in relations between nineteenth-century American medicine and the Paris clinical revolution is John Harley Warner's *Against the Spirit of System,* a prodigious example of original archival work in a largely unexplored area. Warner's exhaustive footnotes serve in themselves as a useful guide to sources on nineteenth-century American medicine. Warner's earlier work, *The Therapeutic Perspective,* and his contribution to Hannaway and La Berge's *Constructing Paris Medicine*—"Paradigm Lost or Paradise Declining? American Physicians and the 'Dead End' of the Paris Clinical School"—will also be of interest to scholars in American history or literature who find themselves at a point of intersection between the humanities and medicine.

I want to mention one primary work, because it seems to me something that everyone with a serious interest in early American literature and social history ought to read sooner or later, whether or not they are specifically interested in medicine as such. This is *The Life of John Collins Warren, M.D., Compiled Chiefly from his Autobiography and Journals* by his son, Edward Warren. John Collins Warren, representing the third generation in a distinguished Boston medical family, was a surgeon, a Harvard professor of medicine, a moving spirit in civic affairs, and a complex and fascinating personality—one of those extraordinary Victorian souls who today seem to us, in their unwearying devotion to duty, their courage under stress, and their unshakable moral integrity, to be almost creatures from a different world. For students of literary Boston, especially, the biography is irreplaceable: the world into which Oliver Wendell Holmes was born in 1809 was the one the reader enters when opening the first page of *The Life of John Collins Warren.* I can imagine no better way of hearing the living voices of its people than following Warren through his long and eventful life. It is long past time that the work was reprinted.

I should also mention that Howard Payson Arnold's memoir of Jonathan Mason Warren is another fascinating source for those interested in Boston literary and medical culture. Its account of Mason's medical studies in Paris, based on a close and sympathetic reading of Mason's Paris journal, gives as vivid an impression of the Trois Frères group as one could wish for. Privately printed in a limited edition, it is today found mostly in rare book depositories and history of medicine libraries. One hopes that it, too, might be reprinted before our new century gets much older.

As for work on Holmes himself, the situation remains—except for one significant study I shall mention in a moment—about where it was over thirty years ago, when Barry Menikoff wrote his extensive bibliographical and critical survey of Holmes scholarship in Rees and Herbert's

Fifteen American Authors Before 1900. The significant study that has just appeared is Peter Gibian's *Oliver Wendell Holmes and the Culture of Conversation,* which begins by noting that Holmes in recent years has virtually dropped off the map of American literary studies. In "losing Holmes," as Gibian quite correctly says, "we have lost a brilliant writer and a provocative thinker," as well as a major figure in the American Renaissance.

The most cursory glance at the table of contents in any recent anthology of American literature will show what Gibian means. A widely-used anthology I have just examined, for instance, shows substantial selections from Philip Freneau, Phillis Wheatley, and Margaret Fuller. Its selections from Walt Whitman, running on page after page, amount to a small anthology in themselves. For Holmes, there is nothing from *The Autocrat of the Breakfast Table* or the later volumes in the Breakfast Table trilogy, nothing from his writings on medicine and science, and nothing from his numerous occasional essays. The thirteen volumes of his collected works have shrunk, in at least this one undergraduate anthology, to four poems, three of which—*Old Ironsides, The Last Leaf,* and *The Chambered Nautilus*—have the advantage of being short, the other of which—*The Wonderful One-Hoss Shay*—has the advantage of being funny. The equivalent in an anthology of Renaissance literature, one supposes, would be a section in which Shakespeare was represented solely by *Blow, Blow, Thou Winter Wind* and *Where the Bee Sucks, There Suck I.*

Nonetheless, the resistance of New England civic and intellectual culture to the raw economic individualism associated with Jacksonian democracy has recently begun to draw the attention of serious scholars. The extended recent period during which authors and works have been added to the literature syllabus for political or ideological reasons rather than on literary grounds seems at last to be drawing to an end. I do not think it too much to expect that there will be a "rediscovery" of literary Boston before long. The representatives of New England literary culture who have managed to hold their places in the anthologies—Emerson, say, or Hawthorne—have done so only by being separated from the intellectual ethos of Holmes and Boston and the Saturday Club and presented as voices speaking in a disembodied "American" register. But Emerson and Hawthorne were, like Holmes and Lowell and Motley, members of the Saturday Club. Emerson, for one, rarely missed a meeting. *The Autocrat of the Breakfast Table* was a product of the same literary culture that gave birth to *The Divinity School Address* and *The Scarlet Letter.* It is only a matter of time, one suspects, before that culture once again becomes an object of serious study.

In *Oliver Wendell Holmes and the Culture of Conversation,* Peter Gibian has drawn on most of the important primary and secondary materials. For my own argument in the preceding chapters, two are especially important: Mark DeWolfe Howe's *The Atlantic Monthly and Its Makers*, and Edward Waldo Emerson's *The Early Years of the Saturday Club*. Van Wyck Brooks's account of Holmes in *The Flowering of New England*, though carrying traces of the condescension that would drive Holmes out of the anthologies after the publication of Vernon Parrington's *Main Currents in American Thought* (1930)—roughly speaking, an attempt to retell the story of American literature and culture from the perspective of what Parrington himself calls "coonskin egalitarianism"—is a solid general or popular introduction. Barrett Wendell's *A Literary History of America*, which in some ways shows a more sophisticated grasp of literary and intellectual history than many works of modern scholarship, has a useful chapter on Holmes. It is not, however, the strongest portion of Wendell's work.

The standard biography of Holmes for many years was John T. Morse's Victorian life-and-letters treatment in two volumes, written by someone who was not only related to Holmes, but who as a child was treated by him during the short period when Holmes was a practicing physician. (His complaint was a catarrh. Holmes prescribed wine of ipecac, syrup of squills, and four drops of laudanum. Morse, then three years old, recovered nicely.) To anyone interested in Holmes's Paris medical studies, volume one of Morse's *Life and Letters of Oliver Wendell Holmes* is particularly valuable for its collection of letters written by Holmes to his parents from Paris. A comparison of these letters with the collection from which Morse was working shows that very little of importance was left out.

The standard modern biography is Eleanor M. Tilton's *Amiable Autocrat: A Biography of Dr. Oliver Wendell Holmes*. In anyone who has done much original research on Holmes, the volume arouses conflicting feelings. Miss Tilton—as she preferred to be called—did not have great narrative gifts, and her biography is an example of the relentless one-thing-after-another mode in which so many academic biographies at midcentury tended to be written. ("The cry of 'man overboard,' caused a furor," she dutifully reports in her account of Holmes's departure for Europe. "Someone tossed a plank over the side and the floundering sailor was speedily hauled up." There is a great deal of this sort of thing.) On the other hand, Miss Tilton was a genuinely great scholar: anyone who goes in depth into the Holmes Collection at Harvard finds, in every folder of materials, in every box of manuscripts, in attachments to innumerable notebooks and letters, that Miss Tilton has already been there, correcting dates, cross-referencing scribbled notes to published works, identifying unknown correspondents. Over the years that I was working with the Holmes Collection, I came to regard Miss Tilton as a friend and guardian angel.

Perhaps Miss Tilton's greatest contribution to the study of Holmes and literary Boston was her monumental *Bibliography of Oliver Wendell Holmes*, begun by Thomas Franklin Currier and completed by her after his death. Though the appendix on "Biography and Criticism" is by now a bit dated, it will remain the indispensable starting-point for scholars interested in contemporary responses to Holmes's writings, as well as the transatlantic cultural milieu out of which they emerge. Where else would one find precise bibliographical references to Edmund Gosse's "An Epistle to Dr. Oliver Wendell Holmes on His Seventy-Fifth Birthday," as it was simultaneously printed in both *The Athenaeum* and *The Critic*, with a separate private printing of 40 copies for friends of Gosse and Holmes? As for Miss Tilton's identifications, listings, and bibliographical descriptions of works published during Holmes's lifetime, they are, in their completeness, thoroughness, and exactitude, beyond praise.

A biography of Holmes that tends not to come up for mention in the standard bibliographical surveys, but that in certain strange ways has a unique value for students of the period, is William Sloane Kennedy's *Oliver Wendell Holmes: Poet, Littérateur, Scientist*, published in 1883, during Holmes's lifetime. Written by someone who was clearly obsessed with Holmes, it veers wildly from extravagant praise for Holmes's writing to barely-disguised anger at his insufficiently "democratic" social attitudes. Holmes and members of his circle ignored the work—though Francis Underwood, who thought it snide and mean-spirited, wanted to write a counter-biography to right the balance, and took some steps towards doing so—and it has tended to be ignored in later scholarship. But Kennedy's narrative, whatever its psychological motivation, contains a wealth of biographical data that cannot be found elsewhere, and does not lack a certain shrewdness in its estimate of Holmes's impact on nineteenth-century American intellectual culture.

I have mentioned Barry Menikoff's survey of Holmes scholarship in Rees and Harbert's *Fifteen American Authors Before 1900* (Madison: University of Wisconsin Press, 1971). Menikoff's treatment of the relevant scholarly resources, and of the course of Holmes criticism in the twentieth century, is thorough and thoughtful, especially strong in its coverage of British reviews and responses to Holmes's work during his lifetime. A special virtue, for readers of the present work, is that Menikoff lists scholarly notes and articles on Holmes's medical writings, many by medical professors or practicing physicians, in a separate section. He does not mention Sir William Osler's wonderfully engaging chapter in *An Alabama Student And Other Essays*, which presents Holmes as "the most successful combination which the world has ever seen of the physician and the man of letters." It is a handsome tribute from one great medical humanist to another.

Though the Countway Medical Library at Harvard contains a wealth of materials related to Holmes's career as a physician and writer, those related to his Paris medical studies are mainly to be found in the Holmes Collection at Houghton Library. The collection is catalogued in very general terms, meaning that scholars seeking specific items concerning Holmes as medical student, practicing physician, or Parkman Professor have to work pretty much by trial and error until they get to know the significance of entries in the bound finding list available in the main reading room. Since the cataloguing is so approximate that there would be no real point to giving shelf and box numbers—many of which, additionally, have been changed in recent years as new accessions have come in—I have simply listed the Holmes Collection as my source. Unless otherwise noted, notes always refer to items in the Houghton repository.

For social and political background on Jacksonian America, I will simply refer the reader to Charles Sellers's exhaustive notes and lengthy bibliographical essay in *The Market Revolution*. Sellers's book has been controversial—I myself disagree strongly with many of its conclusions, as well as the specific concept of "the market" that lies at the center of its analysis—but no one can deny that it is the most comprehensive and learned treatment of its subject yet produced, the work of a scholar who has spent a lifetime mastering the inordinately complex social and political reality of Jacksonian America. To anyone wishing to understand John Haller's *The People's Doctors*, John Harley Warner's discussion of the licensing controversy in *The Therapeutic Perspective*, or, indeed, my own argument about the resistance of the Boston medical community to the forces of Jacksonian economic individualism, *The Market Revolution* is an indispensable resource.

Notes

References to works contained in the thirteen-volume Riverside edition
of Holmes works are to that edition. Information on Holmes titles published independent of that edition are given in full in the "Bibliography."
For reasons explained in the "Note on Sources," references to items in
the Holmes Collection at Harvard have been annotated with the shorthand citation HCHL—"Holmes Collection, Houghton Library." The
text in quotations from Sir Thomas Browne has been modernized. When
possible, I have used shorthand titles for all works contained in the bibliography. Unless otherwise noted, translations from French, German,
and Latin sources are mine.

Preface (pages vii–xvi)

1. Kennedy, *Holmes*: 132–133.
2. Kennedy, *Holmes*: 133.
3. Motley, *Correspondence*: I. 226.
4. *Autocrat*, 1891 preface: iix.
5. HCHL: Phipson to OWH, 24 April 1876.
6. HCHL: Parnell to OWH, 28 August 18?? [ms. illegible].
7. HCHL: Boyd to OWH, 24 July 1874.
8. HCHL: Collier to Oliver Wendell Holmes, Jr., 14 Feb 1931.
9. Holmes's note is to the *American Literary Gazette* for November 15, 1867.
10. Quoted in Houghton, *The Victorian Frame of Mind*: 71.
11. "Paris Medicine: Perspectives Past and Present," in Hannaway and La
Berge, *Constructing Paris Medicine*: 13.
12. "The Medical Profession in Massachusetts," in *Medical Essays*: 364.
13. The term *coupure*, meant to signal a sharp break with a previously dominant system of thought, is associated in French philosophy of science with the
work of Bachelard. For a good account of how the term functions in Bachelard's account of scientific inquiry, see Tiles, *Bachelard: Science and Objectivity*.
(As popularized in the "archaeology" of Foucault, "rupture" has become more
the more common term.) As with the distantly related notion of a "paradigm
shift" in Thomas Kuhn's *Structure of Scientific Revolutions*, such terms are meant

to emphasize that discontinuities are as crucial in the history of thought as the grand continuities dwelt on in an older style of intellectual history. As the philosopher Ian Hacking has remarked, there do periodically occur "sharp mutations in systems of thought," and "these redistributions of ideas establish what later seems inevitable, unquestionable, necessary" (Hacking, *Rewriting the Soul*: 4). In the case of the Paris medical revolution, what would come to seem inevitable would be nothing other than our current notion of disease as the direct result, as Sherwin Nuland puts it, of "specific pathological changes within cells, tissues, and organs, or of disorders in biochemical processes," and the notion that "once these underlying alterations have been identified, they can be shown to have led inevitably to the observed clinical manifestations" (Nuland, *How We Die:* 89).

14. Quoted in Ackerknecht: 56.

15. Gardner, *Old Wine*: 68.

16. The phrase *l'école de la Charité* is Bouillaud's, quoted by Holmes in his Boylston prize "Dissertation on Direct Exploration": 6. A splendid account of the sense of continuity among the successive researchers working at La Charité is L. S. Jacyna's "Au Lit des Malades: A.F. Chomel's Clinic at The Charité, 1828-29."

17. "The Medical Profession in Massachusetts," in *Medical Essays*:353.

18. Sherwin Nuland points out to me that, in terms of our current understanding of *symptom* and *sign*, the phrase "subjective symptomology" is, properly speaking, tautological: a symptom is today understood precisely the subjective manifestation of a pathological state, as opposed to an objective sign, such as might be disclosed by an EKG reading or blood chemistry, that is able to provide evidence of a pathological condition in a person who feels perfectly well. I take Duffin to be using the term to drive home the point that, before the Paris revolution in diagnostic technique, *all* signs of illness were necessarily subjective—i.e., that in the older medical world of Galen theory and practice, the sign/symptom distinction did not exist.

19. "My Early Teachers," in *Medical Essays*: 433.

20. "Border Lines," in *Medical Essays*: 265.

21. "Border Lines," in *Medical Essays*: 251.

22. "Jonathan Edwards," in *Pages from an Old Volume of Life*: 368.

23. Howells, *Literary Friends*: 135.

24. Kennedy, *Holmes*: 237.

25. "Currents and Counter-Currents," in *Medical Essays*:180–181.

26. "What have I rescued from the shelf?
    A Boswell, writing out himself!
    For though he changes dress and name,
    The man beneath is still the same,
    Laughing or sad, by fits and starts,
    One actor in a dozen parts,
    And whatsoe'er the mask may be,
    The voice assures us, *This is he.*"
        —*The Poet at the Breakfast Table*: 350

27. Howells, *Literary Friends*: 146.

1. "My Early Teachers," in *Medical Essays*: 426.
2. "My Early Teachers, in *Medical Essays*: 437.
3. "Homeopathy," in *Medical Essays*: 78.
4. Mott, *Travels*: 39.
5. Urban T. Holmes, *Daily Living in the Twelfth Century*: 137-138.
6. "The Medical Profession in Massachusetts," in *Medical Essays*: 318.
7. Ackerknecht, *Medicine at the Paris Hospital*: 50.
8. Duffin, *To See With a Better Eye*: 27.
9. Duffin, *To See With a Better Eye*: 27.
10. Duffin, *To See With a Better Eye*: 303.
11. King, *Medical World of the Eighteenth Century*: 24–25.
12. Brockliss, "Before the Clinic," in Hannaway and La Berge, *Constructing Paris Medicine*: 71.
13. Morse, *Life and Letters*: I, 151.
14. Ackerknecht, *Medicine at the Paris Hospital*: 32, italics in original.
15. Gardner, *Old Wine*: 19.
16. Gardner, *Old Wine*: 293.
17. Ackerknecht, *Medicine at the Paris Hospital*: 15.
18. Ackerknecht, *Medicine at the Paris Hospital*: 16.
19. Brockliss, "Before the Clinic," in Hannaway and La Berge, *Constructing Paris Medicine*: 92.
20. Hannaway and La Berge, *Constructing Paris Medicine*: 8.
21. Keel, "A Product of the Paris Clinical School?"in Hannaway and La Berge, *Constructing Paris Medicine*: 127.
22. Warren, Edward. *John Collins Warren*: II, 114–115.
23. Gardner, *Old Wine*: 78.
24. "My Early Teachers," in *Medical Essays*: 429.
25. Ackerknecht, *Medicine at the Paris Hospital*: 164.
26. Hannaway and La Berge, *Constructing Paris Medicine*: 6.
27. Duffin, "Laennec and Broussais," in Hannaway and La Berge, *Constructing Paris Medicine*: 266.
28. W. R. Albury, "Corvisart and Broussais,"in Hannaway and La Berge, *Constructing Paris Medicine*: 240.
29. "Border Lines," in *Medical Essays*: 223.
30. King, *The Medical World of the Eighteenth Century*: 272.
31. Duffin, *History of Medicine*: 77.
32. Ackerknecht, *Medicine at the Paris Hospital*: 56.
33. Hannaway and La Berge, *Constructing Paris Medicine*: 24.
34. "Border Lines," in *Medical Essays*: 222.
35. Duffin, *History of Medicine*: 79.
36. Dowling, "Holmes and the Paris Medical Revolution": 64.
37. Warner, "Paradigm Lost or Paradise Declining?" in Hannaway and La Berge, *Constructing Paris Medicine*: 339.
38. Edward Warren, *John Collins Warren*: I, 405.
39. Gardner, *Old Wine*: 68.

40. Morse, *Life and Letters*: I, 151.

41. Arnold, *Memoir*: 308-308.

42. Jones, *Parisian Education of an American Surgeon*: 150.

43. "Border Lines," in *Medical Essays*: 223-24.

44. Duffin, *History of Medicine*: 224.

45. Brockliss, "Before the Clinic," in Hannaway and La Berge, *Constructing Paris Medicine*: 93.

46. Ellis, *A History of the Bladder Stone*: 11.

47. Ellis, *A History of the Bladder Stone*: 10-11.

48. Tilanus, *Surgery A Hundred Years Ago*: 32–45.

49. Tilanus, *Surgery A Hundred Years Ago*: 32–45.

50. Tilanus, *Surgery A Hundred Years Ago*: 32–45.

51. Nuland, *How We Die*: 146.

52. Jones, *Parisian Education of an American Surgeon*: 248.

53. King, *Medical World of the Eighteenth Century*: 318.

54. Tilanus, *Surgery A Hundred Years Ago*: 46–47.

55. Jones, *Parisian Education of an American Surgeon*: 236.

56. Jones, *Parisian Education of an American Surgeon*: 186.

57. "My Early Teachers," in *Medical Essays*: 433.

58. Jones, *Parisian Education of an American Surgeon*: 119.

59. Jones, *Parisian Education of an American Surgeon*: 119.

60. Arnold, *Memoir*: 191.

61. Edward Warren, *John Collins Warren*: I, 334.

62. Edward Warren, *John Collins Warren*: II, 299.

2. *The School of La Charité (pages 28–54)*

1. Morse, *Life and Letters*: I, 89.

2. Gardner, *Old Wine*: 100.

3. Holmes's own recollections of life in the Latin Quarter bear little resemblance to Gibson's somewhat dour memories of filthy streets and crowded houses ("so high, old-fashioned, and gloomy," Gibson goes on in the passage just quoted, "as to resemble jails, or penitentiaries, and nearly shut out the light of heaven"). This was probably because his own lodgings at 55 rue M. Le Prince, only a few steps from the Luxembourg Gardens, were spacious and airy—he was on the fourth floor (third in the French style of counting), with windows looking out on the rue Vaugirard—and very centrally located in relation to the places he would visit most frequently, the École de Médicine itself, the Hôtel Dieu, La Pitié and the Clamart, and the Café Procope, on the rue de l'Ancienne Comèdie. Gibson, *Rambles in Europe*: 65.

4. A vivid sense of how forbidding Paris was for most newly-arrived foreign students can be gotten from Meding's introduction: "Quand on entre dans une grande ville comme Paris, que l'on n'y connaît point d'amis assez intimes ou assez serviables pour vous attendre au débarcadère ou dans la cour des Messageries, et pour vous servier de cicérone, on ressent une impression indéfinissable. Paris est un grand désert peuplé, on y est seul en compagnie." (Meding: I, 19).

The real name of "Henri" Meding was Heinrich Ludwig Meding. He was a German medical student and member of the *Sociéte medicale allemande* in Paris, for whose recently-arrived members he had earlier written several shorter German versions of the same work.

5. HCHL. This occurs in an unpublished talk given by Holmes to the Boston Society for Medical Improvement on November 8, 1841. For a short description, see Currier and Tilton: 435.

6. Jones, *Parisian Education of an American Surgeon*: 174.

7. See Dowling, "Holmes and the Paris Medical Revolution."

8. Bouillaud, quoted by Holmes in *Boylston Prize Dissertations*: 255.

9. HCHL: "Leçons de M. Chomel."

10. HCHL: " Leçons de M. Chomel."

11. "As I was desirous of learning to speak French as soon and as thoroughly as possible, I kept aloof to a certain degree from all Americans, and took my meals with French and Swiss medical and law students. The result of these arrangements was that though living near him I rarely saw Mason, save when we accidentally met as neighbors." Arnold, *Memoir of Jonathan Mason Warren, M.D.*: 268.

12. Arnold, *Memoir*: 72.

13. Jones, *Parisian Education of an American Surgeon*: 7.

14. Morse, *Life and Letters*: I, 102.

15. Morse, *Life and Letters*: I, 148.

16. Jacyna, "'Au lit des malades,'": 423.

17. Jacyna, "'Au lit des malades,'": 425.

18. James Jackson, Sr., *Memoir*: 114.

19. James Jackson, Sr., *Memoir*: 114–115.

20. HCHL: "Louis Clinical Lectures 1834."

21. *Darstellungen und Ansichten zur Vergleichung der Medizin in Frankreich, England und Deutschland.* Ackerknecht: 90.

22. "The Medical Profession in Massachusetts," in *Medical Essays*: 353.

23. Holmes, *Boylston Prize Dissertations* ("Dedicated to P. Cha. A. Louis, Doctor in Medicine in the Faculties of Paris and St. Petersburg, President of the Societé Médicale d'Observation, etc. In the recollection of his invaluable instructions and unvarying kindness"): 250.

24. Holmes, *Boylston Prize Dissertations*: 254.

25. Buchan, *Domestic Medicine*: 131–132.

26. Ackerknecht, *Medicine at the Paris Hospital*: 87.

27. Ackerknecht, *Medicine at the Paris Hospital*: 91.

28. Laennec, *De l'auscultation médiate*: I, 17. "Sa voix semble sortir directement de la poitrine et passer toute entière par le canal central du cylindre."

29. Osler, "Elisha Bartlett," in *An Alabama Student*: 111.

30. Laennec, *De l'auscultation médiate*: I, 21.

31. Dubos, *The White Plague*: 5.

32. Duffin, *To See With a Better Eye*: 157.

33. Laennec, *De l'auscultation médiate*: I, 23.

34. Laennec, *De l'auscultation médiate*: I, 60.

35. Laennec, *De l'auscultation médiate*: I, 60.

36. Laennec, *De l'auscultation médiate*: I, 61.

37. Dubos, *The White Plague*: 89.

38. Holmes, *Boylston Prize Dissertations*: 257.

39. Holmes, *Boylston Prize Dissertations*: 269.

40. See Haller, *The People's Doctors*.

41. Morse, *Life and Letters*: I, 108.

42. Jacyna, "'Au lit des malades,'": 433.

43. Jacyna, "'Au lit des malades,'": 435.

44. Jones, *Parisian Education of an American Surgeon*: 183.

45. James Jackson, Sr., *Memoir*: 111.

46. Jacyna, "'Au lit des malades,'": 433.

47. "The Young Practitioner," in *Medical Essays*: 375.

48. Dubos, *The White Plague*: 59.

49. "The Young Practitioner," in *Medical Essays*: 387–388.

50. "The Young Practitioner," in *Medical Essays*: 389.

51. Warner, *The Therapeutic Perspective*: 280.

52. Broussais, *Examen des doctriens médicales*: 648.

53. Broussais, *Examen des doctriens médicales*: 717. Italics in original.

54. Broussais, *Examen des doctriens médicales*: 718.

55. Anne La Berge and Caroline Hannaway, "Paris Medicine: Perspectives Past and Present," in *Constructing Paris Medicine*: 17. John Harley Warner has also noted the appreciation of theatricality among American medical students in Paris: "The rhetoric Americans used in describing such clinical instruction commonly included vividly detailed attention to the physical staging of the room, how the orator's voice sounded, how he dressed, and the character his physical presence conveyed. Such reports betrayed an underlying sense of clinical instruction as spectacle, a relished sense of the theatricality of seeing the medical lions perform." "Paradigm Lost or Paradise Declining? American Physicians and the 'Dead End' of the Paris Clinical School," in Hannaway and La Berge, *Constructing Paris Medicine*: 349.

56. Ackerknecht, *Medicine at the Paris Hospital*: 79.

57. Arnold, *Memoir*: 83–84.

58. "My Early Teachers," in *Medical Essays*: 431.

59. James Jackson, Sr., *Memoir*: 163.

60. Ackerknecht, *Medicine at the Paris Hospital*: 101.

61. Duffin, *To See With a Better Eye*: 253.

62. "Border Lines," in *Medical Essays*: 211.

63. Duffin, *To See With a Better Eye*: 32.

64. Duffin, *To See With a Better Eye*, 163-166.

65. Duffin, *To See With a Better Eye*: 50.

66. Holmes, *Boylston Prize Dissertations*: 267.

67. Holmes, *Boylston Prize Dissertations*: 268.

68. HCHL: "Andral Internal Pathology 1833"

69. HCHL: "Andral Internal Pathology 1833"

70. HCHL: "Andral Internal Pathology 1833"

71. HCHL: Bartlett to Holmes, 6 February 1844.

72. Warner, *Against the Spirit of System*: 175.

73. HCHL: Bartlett to Holmes, 6 February 1844.

74. Osler, "Elisha Bartlett," in *An Alabama Student*: 134.

75. James Jackson, Sr., *Memoir*: 126–127.

3. *The Clinic of Doctor Louis (pages 55–82)*

1. Osler, "Influence of Louis on American Medicine," in *An Alabama Student*: 198.

2. Bowditch, *Brief Memories of Louis*: 27.

3. "My Early Teachers," in *Medical Essays*: 431.

4. "My Early Teachers," in *Medical Essays*: 436.

5. Arnold, *Memoir*: 109.

6. Tocqueville, *Democracy in America*: II, 237.

7. Anderson, "Henry James's Cultural Office": 27.

8. James Jackson, Sr., *Memoir*: 28–29

9. King: 230. King is especially good on the role of the guild in protecting a trade or profession against the indiscriminate forces of the market: "In certain trades or professions unrestrained competition might depress all standards. Poorly trained workers might flood the market with shoddy goods or incompetent services. The conscientious and well-qualified workers would suffer and so would the general public. The remedy was the guild. An organized group received from the ruling authority a charter granting a strict monopoly in certain goods or services. In return the guild guaranteed a high standard of quality. Society as a whole benefitted from the improved standards" (230–231).

10. Ackerknecht, *Medicine at the Paris Hospital*: 25.

11. "His honest, unambitious parents, destined their son to follow the trade of a blacksmith, the occupation of his father. By some accident his father, although illiterate, possessed all the books of the village, which happened to be, a *Treatise of Hippocrates*, *The Country Mason*, and *The Poor Folk's Doctor*. Having learnt these works by heart, Velpeau—the son—was frequently called upon to treat the sick in the neighborhood. . . . [A local doctor is astonished at his knowledge, and sends him to Tours to study.] Time . . . at length brought him to Paris; and in a public *Concour* he gained the situation of *interne*, or house-physician, of the hospital St. Louis. Here he was at least exempted from the necessity of sleeping in a garret. . . . His last effort was for the Chair of Clinical Surgery against the celebrated Lisfranc, Panson, the elder—and Blandin. In this attempt with such distinguished rivals, he bore away the palm." Gardner, *Old Wine in New Bottles*: 80.

12. Gardner, *Old Wine*: 81.

13. Gibson, *Rambles in Europe*: 64.

14. James Jackson, Sr., *Memoir*: 81.

15. Tocqueville, *Democracy in America*: II, 247–248.

16. James Jackson, Sr., *Memoir*: 80.

17. James Jackson, Sr., *Memoir*: 101–102.

18. James Jackson, Sr., *Memoir*: 175.

19. Osler, "Elisha Bartlett," in *An Alabama Student*: 128.

20. Tocqueville, *Democracy in America*: II, 336.

21. On a visit to Paris in 1845, Elisha Bartlett, who had not studied with Louis during his own earlier medical training, made a point of seeking him out. "I have seen a good deal of Louis," he reported in a letter to a friend, "who has been very civil and attentive. I dined with him soon after my arrival. . . . I never see him that he does not speak of young Jackson—*ce pauvre Jackson*, as he calls hm. He told me, with a great deal of feeling, that Jackson, the last night he spent in Paris, wrote him a letter from his hotel, which was moistened with his tears, and that he thought Jackson was almost as much attached to him as to his father." Osler: 123.

22. "My Early Teachers," in *Medical Essays*: 425.

23. "My Early Teachers," in *Medical Essays*: 433.

24. Rothstein, *American Physicians in the 19th Century*: 37.

25. An interesting aspect of Rush's relationship to Jeffersonian ideology is that Jefferson himself, though a steadfast supporter of the abstract political doctrines enunciated during the Jacobin ascendancy in the French Revolution, was an opponent of speculative systems in medicine: "The adventurous physician . . . substitutes presumption for knowledge. From the scanty field of what is known, he launches into the boundless region of what is unknown. He establishes for his guide some fanciful theory of corpuscular attraction, of chemical agency, of mechanical powers, of stimuli, of irritability accumulated or exhausted, of depletion by the lancet & repletion by mercury, or some other ingenious dream, which lets him into all nature's secrets at short hand." (Rothstein: 42).

26. "Currents and Counter-Currents," in *Medical Essays*:180.

27. "Homeopathy," in *Medical Essays*: 92.

28. See O'Brien, *The Long Affair*.

29. King, *Medical World of the Eighteenth Century*: 149.

30. King, *Medical World of the Eighteenth Century*: 148.

31. King, *Medical World of the Eighteenth Century*: 223–224.

32. King, *Medical World of the Eighteenth Century*: 148.

33. Warner, *The Therapeutic Perspective*: 91-92.

34. "Currents and Counter-Currents," in *Medical Essays*:181-182.

35. Warner, *The Therapeutic Perspective*: 18.

36. Kaufman, *Homeopathy*: 2.

37. Kaufman, *Homeopathy*: 2.

38. Rothstein, *American Physicians in the 19th Century*: 48.

39. Rothstein, *American Physicians in the 19th Century*: 46.

40. "Scholastic and Bedside Teaching," in *Medical Essays*: 293.

41. "Border Lines," in *Medical Essays*: 254-255.

42. Ricord, immortalized by Holmes as "the Voltaire of pelvic literature" for the cynical view of human nature he had learned from listening to his patients explain their venereal diseases, had also been Mason Warren's teacher in Paris. Mason's letters to John Collins Warren suggest how incontestable was the efficacy of the mercury treatment of syphilis in Ricord's view: "In the first place from numerous experiments by inoculation . . . he goes a great way to prove that the viruses of chancre and gonorrhea are incapable of producing each other and that when we find secondary symptoms arising from an *ecoulement de l'uretre* we

may infer that there is a chancre within. . . . Ricord also thinks that the virus of the chancre becomes *nulle* when the constitution is well under the influence of mercury and that secondary ulcers are not capable of producing the disease" (Jones: 211–121).

43. Sartin and Perry, "From mercury to penicillin": 255–61.

44. "Border Lines," in *Medical Essays*: 255.

45. Rothstein, *American Physicians in the 19th Century*: 51.

46. Warren, *John Collins Warren*: II, 200.

47. "Border Lines,"in *Medical Essays*: 254.

48. Rothstein, *American Physicians in the 19th Century*: 52.

49. "Currents and Counter-Currents," in *Medical Essays*: 193.

50. James Jackson, Sr., *Memoir*: 177–178.

51. James Jackson, Sr., *Memoir*: 177–178.

52. James Jackson, Sr., *Memoir*: 167.

53. "Puerperal Fever," in *Medical Essays*: 124.

54. Ackerknecht, *Medicine at the Paris Hospital*: 48.

55. "Border Lines in Medical Science," in *Medical Essays*:180. Holmes is describing the overall movement studied in John Harley Warner's *The Therapeutic Perspective*, which traces the shift from a concept of health as a "natural" balance to a "normal" state: "To the extent that words reflect and mold thinking, this alteration in clinical language marked an important change in cognition. The shift in the way physicians thought about disease—from a disruption of a natural balance to a deviation from fixed norms—had fundamental implications for medical theory, epistemology, and professional identity." Warner, *The Therapeutic Perspective*: 91.

56. James Jackson, Sr., *Memoir*: 95.

57. "Que le lecteur sache encore, car il faut qu'il le sache, que je n'ai vu que deux fois l'illustre Laënnec, pour quelques minutes chaque fois; que je n'ai jamais assisté a ses leçons; que le seul médecin que j'aie entendu professer la pathologie interne est M. Broussais; et qu'il s'explique pourquoi M. Broussais répète en vingt endroits, ou donne à entendre, que je suis l'élève et l'élève obséquieux de Laënnec, si ce n'est pour m'avilir aux yeux du lecteur et appuyer une critique dont il n'a pu se dissimuler l'impuissance." Louis, *Examen de l'éxamen*: 5.

58. Louis, *Examen de l'éxamen*: 81–82.

59. "My Early Teachers," in *Medical Essays*: 432.

60. James Jackson, Sr., *Memoir*: 73.

61. James Jackson, Sr., *Memoir*: 74.

62. James Jackson, Sr., *Memoir*: 98.

63. In 1837, for instance, John Collins Warren would head a committee formed in response to an outbreak of spotted fever in Massachusetts. "'Before the appearance of this pamphlet,' says Dr. Alden, in his Address to the Massachusetts Medical Society in 1838, 'the treatment had been, in many cases, empirical, and of course, in those instances, prejudicial. Active stimulants, opium, brandy, and steaming, were too often indiscriminately used; and it was the opinion of intelligent and cautious observers, that not a few of the individuals attacked died of the remedies rather than the disease'." *Life of John Collins Warren*, I: 95.

64. John Harley Warner notes that, in individual cases, the phrase became a kind of shorthand meant to declare familiarity, if not agreement with, the teachings of the Paris school: "In conscious acknowledgment of the term's partially French parentage, American physicians widely adopted the phrase *médecine expectante* to describe the posture." *The Therapeutic Perspective*: 185.

65. "The Medical Profession in Massachusetts," in *Medical Essays*: 351.

66. "My Early Teachers," in *Medical Essays*: 435.

67. Holmes always delighted in pointing out that Cotton Mather, whose Puritan grandiosity he loved to puncture, had to be taught the practice of smallpox inoculation by his own Negro servant: "But now they learn this way: people take juice of *small-pox* and *cutty-skin* and put in a Drop; then by an' by a little sicky, sick; then very few little things like *small-pox*; and nobody dy of it; and nobody have small-pox any more. Thus, in *Africa,* where the poor creatures dy of the *small-pox* like Rotten Sheep, a merciful God has taught them an Infallible preservative." "The Medical Profession in Massachusetts,' in *Medical Essays*: 363.

68. "Preface" to *Medical Essays*: vi.

69. Bigelow, "Self-Limited Diseases," in *Nature and Disease*: 4.

70. Bigelow, "Self-Limited Diseases,"in *Nature and Disease*: 34.

71. The passages are printed as they appear, no doubt showing the unfamiliarity of local compositors with French orthography and accents, in "On Self-Limited Diseases," in *Nature and Disease*: 19.

72. Bigelow, "Self-Limited Diseases,"in *Nature and Disease*: 31-32.

73. Bigelow, "Self-Limited Diseases,"in *Nature and Disease*: 35.

74. This was almost certainly a lesson made vivid, for Holmes and his Boston companions, by Louis's reputation as someone whose abilities in stethoscopic exploration surpassed even those of the great Laennec. This was especially true in cases where the patient had symptoms consistent with the early stages of tuberculosis, which was notoriously hard to distinguish even from such ordinary conditions as susceptibility to bronchial infection or what we should now attribute to allergic reaction. A persistent cough might be either a mere nuisance or a death warrant. Gardner's *Old Wine in New Bottles* contains a scene that illustrates, better than anything else I know from this period, what Holmes means by the relief from exaggerated fears afforded by the knowledge of a competent physician. The patient in this case is Gardner's cousin Ellen, who has traveled to Paris solely and specifically to consult Louis:

> Louis is the most eminent living physician, who attends to diseases of the chest, and his works are translated into every tongue. . . . Louis is tall and commanding in person, though somewhat stooping. His face, formerly quite full, is now rather thin, and deeply marked with thought; an expression which is increased by his use of spectacles—quite uncommon among the Paris physicians. His hair, formerly light, is now silvered over. . . . The meeting took place; the important examination which had been sought at such a distance, so long, so anxiously, was over. "Madam, there is no disease of the lungs." Was it not worth the labor and expense of a voyage across the Atlantic? (276–277)

75. "Homeopathy," *Medical Essays*: 71.

76. Bigelow, "Treatment of Disease," in *Nature and Disease*: 71.

77. Bigelow, "Treatment of Disease," in *Nature and Disease*: 69–70.

78. "Currents and Counter-Currents," in *Medical Essays*: 186.

79. "The Young Practitioner," in *Medical Essays*: 380.

80. Bigelow, "Treatment of Disease,"in *Nature and Disease*: 65.

81. Bigelow, "Self-Limited Diseases," in *Nature and Disease*: 37.

82. Arnold, *Memoir*: 276.

83. Paley, *Natural Theology*: 274.

84. See Smith, "Gerhard's Distinction between Typhoid and Typhus."

85. Tocqueville, *Democracy in America*, I: 333.

86. Quoted in Tyack, *George Ticknor*: 174.

87. Quoted in Jacyna, "Au lit des malades": 420–449.

88. "Broussais' case was by no means the only one in the history of medicine in which the fate of a scientific idea was profoundly influenced by the political convictions of its promoter. Benjamin Rush, a kind of American Broussais, stated repeatedly, and in our opinion rightly, that his opinions on yellow fever would have found much less opposition had he not been a political exponent of the then unpopular left." Ackerknecht, *Medicine at the Paris Hospital*: 78. Ackerknecht is especially good on the political basis of Broussais's appeal to French medical students: "To them Broussais was often the incarnation of medical progress, because this old soldier of the Revolution, this fierce rebel against the king's Faculty, this outspoken materialist, was the living symbol of their dreams of freedom and justice. How could a man who was so right in politics, a field obviously easy for everybody to understand, not be right in the somewhat more complex field of medicine?" *Medicine at the Paris Hospital*, 76.

89. Kohl's chapter on "The Jacksonian World" in *The Politics of Individualism* is especially good on the common view of Jackson as a "second Jefferson," as when he cites an article from a Jacksonian newspaper in 1834: "This *putting down* is but a repetition of the *old story* of 1798. It is not Jackson that is personally meant,—it is *democracy*, and the Constitution, *personified* and slandered in him, as they were personified and slandered in Jefferson thirty years ago, and as every man who holds the same opinions will be slandered" (Kohl, 40).

90. Tocqueville, *Democracy in America*: 2:336. Paris medical students often remarked on the absence, in Paris, of an American pressure to perfect conformity of public opinion. Thus, for instance, Augustus Gardner: "Is the Frenchman a bondman? Certainly not. In many respects indeed he is freer than my countryman. He is not depressed by the surveillance of public opinion, which, though often a salutary check, is sometimes . . . the most vexatious of tyrants. . . . Though this odious despotism of the public, which spares not even one's own castle, does not possess the power of actual imprisonment, it notwithstanding imposes heavy bail." Gardner, *Old Wine in New Bottles*: 101.

91. Tocqueville, *Democracy in America*: 2: 336.

92. Quoted in Warner, *The Therapeutic Perspective*: 217.

93. Warner, *The Therapeutic Perspective*: 134.

94. "Image a hundred horses, each with two prancing hoofs high poised in air . . . ; a hundred mountebanks, chattering and gibbering their inconceivable jargon, some habited as generals, some as Turks,—some offering their nostrums in the impressive habit of an Armenian Jew, and others rolling head-over-heels upon a stage, and presenting a dose with the grin of Grimaldi. We stopped more

than once in our progress to watch . . . : the poor victim was cajoled and coaxed into believing that none of women born could ever taste of evil more, if he would but trust to the only true, sure, and certain specific." Frances Trollope, *Paris and the Parisians in 1835*: I, 123.

95. Holmes, "Currents and Counter-Currents," in *Medical Essays*: 186.

96. Emerson, *Journals*: IV, 95.

97. Parker, *The Nebraska Question*: 29.

98. Tocqueville, *Democracy in America*: II, 44.

99. Tocqueville, *Democracy in America*: I, 54.

100. Quoted in Tyack, *George Ticknor*: 174.

101. Emerson, *Journals*: IV, 242.

102. Quoted in Tyack, *George Ticknor*: 81.

103. Howard Payson Arnold, *Memoir*: 215.

104. "Currents and Counter-Currents," in *Medical Essays*: 183.

105. HCHL: OWH to Emerson, 4 April 1856.

4. *The Spirit of Paris (pages 83–109)*

1. "Currents and Counter-Currents," in *Medical Essays*: 203.

2. "Preface to the New Edition." *Medical Essays*: xv.

3. Tilton, *Amiable Autocrat*: 255.

4. "The great triumph of the microscope as applied to anatomy has been in the resolution of the organs and the tissues into their simple constituent anatomical elements. It has taken up general anatomy where Bichat left it. He had succeeded in reducing the structural language of nature to syllables, if you will permit me to use so bold an image. The microscopic observers who have come after him have analyzed these into *letters*, as we may call them—the simple elements by the combination of which Nature spells out successively tissues, which are her syllables, organs which are her words, systems which are her chapters, and so goes on from the simple to the complex, until she binds up in one living whole that wondrous volume of power and wisdom which we call the human body." "Border Lines in Medical Knowledge." *Medical Essays*: 228.

5. W. R. Albury. "Corvisart and Broussais," in Hannaway and La Berge, *Constructing Paris Medicine*: 225.

6. Osler, "Elisha Bartlett," in *An Alabama Student*: 130.

7. Paley, *Natural Theology*: 250.

8. Paley, *Natural Theology*: 231.

9. Paley, *Natural Theology*: 239.

10. Gardner, *Old Wine*: 270.

11. Paley, *Natural Theology*: 295

12. "Border Lines,"in *Medical Essays*: 251.

13. "Currents and Counter-Currents," in *Medical Essays*: 180

14. "Medical Libraries," in *Medical Essays*: 417.

15. "Border Lines," in *Medical Essays*: 220.

16. "Currents and Counter-Currents," in *Medical Essays*: 183. The occasion of these remarks was William J. Walker's treatise on the management of com-

pound fractures—that is, a broken leg in which a portion of the bone has broken through the skin. Lest Holmes seem foolishly effusive here, it should be noted that, in the days before antisepsis and germ theory, a compound fracture was almost automatically a reason for amputating the leg. Once the skin had been broken, any attempt to set the bone and let the fracture heal was normally to invite either a later amputation for advanced gangrene—much more dangerous to a badly weakened patient—or death by septicemia. Only when Lister had perfected his system of antiseptic dressings, which had to be managed so fastidiously that many physicians refused to employ them, did it become safe to turn a compound fracture over to the natural healing process.

17. Paley, *Natural Theology*: 293.

18. "The Medical Profession in Massachusetts," in *Medical Essays*: 365.

19. "Border Lines," in *Medical Essays*: 270.

20. "The Medical Profession in Massachusetts ," in *Medical Essays*: 367.

21. "The Medical Profession in Massachusetts," in *Medical Essays*: 331.

22. "The Medical Profession in Massachusetts," in *Medical Essays*: 333.

23. "The Medical Profession in Massachusetts," in *Medical Essays*:360.

24. "The Medical Profession in Massachusetts," in *Medical Essays*: 365.

25. "Puerperal Fever," in *Medical Essays*: 163.

26. Osler, "Oliver Wendell Holmes," in *An Alabama Student*: 66.

27. Quoted in King, *The Medical World of the Eighteenth Century*: 318.

28. "Puerperal Fever," in *Medical Essays*: 162–63.

29. Osler, "Oliver Wendell Holmes," in *An Alabama Student*: 65.

30. "Puerperal Fever," in *Medical Essays*: 132.

31. "Puerperal Fever," in *Medical Essays*: 137.

32. "Puerperal Fever," in *Medical Essays*: 103.

33. "Puerperal Fever," in *Medical Essays*: 107.

34. "Puerperal Fever," in *Medical Essays*: 129.

35. "Puerperal Fever," in *Medical Essays*: 141.

36. Tilton, *Amiable Autocrat*: 174.

37. Tilton, *Aimiable Autocrat*: 174. A full account of the controversy with Meigs and Hodge is given by Tilton, 172–176.

38. The subject arises when his parents are urging him to come home, not least because their own financial resources are being stretched by his extended stay in Paris. "Do not," Holmes wrote them, "be distressed with imaginary evils—put on a little of the Roman spirit and above all if any pecuniary considerations disturb your quiet, remember that Dr. Channing is said to have been years in debt for his European residence and that I am who am worth a hundred of him may pay my debts from my professorship." Tilton, *Aimiable Autocrat*: 131.

39. E.g., Holmes's case notes on one W. Lee, who first came to see him on March 18th, 1843:

> Called at office and said he had not been well for a fortnight. Symptoms had nothing definite about them.—In the same house with him are two persons one sick with typhoid fever and erysipelas, the other with a very bad sore throat.—I thought he would be better for a good clearing out—so ordered
>
> Pil. Cathart. Comp. No. l iii at night
> In morning if no operation 3 iii. Infus. Leuni comp. Diète.

—the next day Sunday I did not see him.

Monday 20th he called—felt better after medicine but has had a redness appear on nose with great tenderness and swelling. This has diminished, but it is still very obvious. P.[ulse] 88 T.[ongue] not bad—no remarkable symptoms that I can ascertain.

Quin. Sulph. Gr. J every 3 hours. Animal food.

Tuesday 21st. Has taken 5 pills. Redness, tenderness, swelling still less than yesterday. P.[ulse] 72.

Sunday March 25th—Mr. Lee had no further trouble from his nose in a day or two—there were in the house when he was attacked a case of typhoid fever and erysipelas and two very bad cases of sore throat. I think this may probably have been a case of erysipelas which aborted, perhaps on account of the powerful cathartic given just before it was coming on." (HCHL)

40. Quoted in Tilton, *Aimiable Autocrat,* 175. Tilton however mistranscribes Bartlett's sentence as "How the hungry heads of that Hydra keep shouting out!"

41. W. S. Kennedy, *Holmes*: 132–133.

42. "Puerperal Fever," in *Medical Essays*: 109.

43. "Puerperal Fever," in *Medical Essays*: 108.

44. "Puerperal Fever," in *Medical Essays*: 112.

45. "Puerperal Fever," in *Medical Essays*: 116.

46. "Puerperal Fever," in *Medical Essays*: 103.

47. "Puerperal Fever," in *Medical Essays*: 120.

48. "Puerperal Fever," in *Medical Essays*: 105.

49. "Puerperal Fever," in *Medical Essays*: 125.

50. "The Contagiousness of Puerperal Fever," in *Medical Essays*: 124.

51. For an extended account of the theory of internal or dramatic audience, as well as *double énonciation*, see Dowling, *The Epistolary Moment.*

52. "Preface." *Professor at the Breakfast Table*: x.

53. "Puerperal Fever," in *Medical Essays*: 128.

54. The original series consisted of three lectures, collectively called by Holmes "Scientific Mysticism": (1) Astrology and Alchemy, (2) Medical Delusions, and (3) Homeopathy. Eleanor Tilton's chronological list shows the series being delivered in 1841-42. The latter two were combined, with editing, into the version published as *Homeopathy and Its Kindred Delusions* in Holmes's *Medical Essays.*

55. Holmes gave up private medical practice in 1849, and at Harvard was dependent on student fees for his income. In collaboration with Jacob Bigelow, Edward Reynolds, and David Humphreys Storer, he had in 1838 founded the Tremont School, in which private clinical instruction was given to medical students during the summer months. His supplementary income from this enterprise depended on student fees as well. He would have no regular salary until President Eliot reformed Harvard Medical School in the 1870s.

56. Norton, C.E., ed. *Correspondence of Carlyle and Emerson*: I: 326.

57. Norton, C.E., ed. *Correspondence of Carlyle and Emerson*: I: 137.

58. Norton, C.E., ed. *Correspondence of Carlyle and Emerson*: I: 132.

59. "Homeopathy," in *Medical Essays*: 43.

60. "Homeopathy," in *Medical Essays*: 44.

61. "Homeopathy," in *Medical Essays*: 53.

62. "Homeopathy," in *Medical Essays*: 55.

63. "Homeopathy," in *Medical Essays*: 75.

64. "Currents and Counter-Currents," 185.

65. "Homeopathy," in *Medical Essays*: 70–71.

66. King, *Medical World of the Eighteenth Century*: 36.

67. Haller, *The People's Doctors*: 53.

68. "Medical Libraries," in *Medical Essays*: 410.

69. Quoted in Haller, *The People's Doctors*: 26.

70. Quoted in Rothstein, *American Physicians in the 19th Century*: 148–149.

71. Quoted in Rothstein, *American Physicians in the 19th Century*: 135. As Haller points out, however, the botanical movement was scarcely less aggressive in its treatment than the "regular" physicians who continued heroic practice: "Ironically, neither the regulars nor the botanics were ready to accept the implications of Jacob Bigelow's lecture 'On Self-Limited Diseases' in 1835. Except for the homeopaths, whom both regulars and Thomsonians castigated in the worst terms, most healers aggressively assaulted disease, willingly attacking maladies with formidable armamentaria of medicines and procedures. While the regulars fought disease with an arsenal that included phlebotomy, mercury, blistering, antimony, and opium, the botanic was armed with a similar assortment of herb-based pukes and purges. Like the regular, the grass-roots botanic was prepared to continue with his regimen or course until the disease—or the patient—succumbed." *The People's Doctors*, 30.

72. Quoted in Kaufman, *Homeopathy*: 23.

73. Daniel H. Whitney. *The Family Physician*: 1.

74. Whitney, *The Family Physician*: 444.

75. Whitney, *The Family Physician*: 444–445.

76. Whitney, *The Family Physician*: 445.

77. Quoted in Rothstein, *American Physicians in the 19th Century*: 123.

78. Quoted in Rothstein, *American Physicians in the 19th Century*: 145.

79. Quoted in Haller, *The People's Doctors*: 132.

80. Quoted in Haller, *The People's Doctors*: 98.

81. "Homeopathy," in *Medical Essays*: 39

82. "Homeopathy and Its Kindred Delusions," in *Medical Essays*: 97. Holmes is of course using "clown" in its literary or Shakespearean sense, meaning a rustic or peasant, and by association as (OED) "implying ignorance, crassness, or rude manners."

83. Kaufman. *Homeopathy*: 29.

84. Quoted in Rothstein, *American Physicians in the 19th Century*: 160.

85. "Those kind friends who suggest to a person suffering from a tedious complaint, that he 'had better try Homeopathy,' are apt to enforce their suggestion by adding that 'at any rate it can do no harm.' This may or may not be true as regards the individual. But it always does very great harm to the community to encourage ignorance, error, or deception in a profession which deals with the life and health of our fellow creatures." *Medical Essays*: 1.

86. "Currents and Counter-Currents," in *Medical Essays*: 175.

87. "Currents and Counter-Currents," in *Medical Essays*: 207.

88. Holmes invokes Arnold's phrase, which occurs in the title of one of the lectures Arnold gave in America, in pointing out the similarities between the views of Arnold and Emerson. He quotes Emerson on the subject: "Shall we judge a country by the majority, or by the minority? By the minority, surely." Then Holmes: "Here we have the doctrine of the 'saving remnant,' which have since recognized in Mr. Matthew Arnold's well-remembered lecture. Our republican philosopher is clearly enough outspoken on this matter of the *vox populi*. 'Leave this hypocritical prating about the masses. Masses are rude, lame, unmade, pernicious in their demands, and need not to be flattered, but to be schooled. I wish not to concede anything to them, but to tame, drill, divide, and break them up, and draw individuals out of them'." *Ralph Waldo Emerson*: 236.

89. "Medical Libraries," in *Medical Essays*: 408.

5. *Religio Medici (pages 110–135)*

1. Quoted in Houghton, *The Victorian Frame of Mind*: 75.
2. Quoted in Houghton, *The Victorian Frame of Mind*: 73.
3. *Poet at the Breakfast Table*: 338.
4. "Medical Libraries," in *Medical Essays*: 417.
5. *Autocrat of the Breakfast Table*: 266.
6. *Professor at the Breakfast Table*: 113.
7. *Professor at the Breakfast Table*: 10–11.
8. *Poet at the Breakfast Table*: 249.
9. For an excellent treatment of this aspect of Holmes's literary achievement, see Peter Gibian, *Oliver Wendell Holmes and the Culture of Conversation*.
10. Osler, "Elisha Bartlett," in *An Alabama Student*: 119.
11. *Autocrat of the Breakfast Table*: 20.
12. *Autocrat of the Breakfast Table*: 22.
13. See Pocock, *The Machiavellian Moment*; Kerber, *Federalists in Dissent*; and Dowling, *Literary Federalism*.
14. *Autocrat of the Breakfast Table*: 23.
15. For background, see Bailyn, *The Ideological Origins of the American Revolution*, and Wood, *The Creation of the American Republic*.
16. Quoted in Tyack, *George Ticknor*: 28.
17. Tyack, *George Ticknor*: 176.
18. Haller, *The People's Doctors*: 53.
19. "The breakfast proceeds in sombre silence," says Mrs. Trollope of one such boarding house, "save that sometimes a parrot, and sometimes a canary bird, ventures to utter a timid note. When it is finished, the gentleman hurry to their occupations, and the quiet ladies mount the stairs, some to the first, some to the second, and some to the third stories, in an inverse proportion to the number of dollars paid."After an early afternoon dinner, the husband again hurries off to his business, the wife does an errand or two, and then "re-enters the cold heartless atmosphere in which she dwells." *Domestic Manners of the Americans*: 220. Such passages represent Trollope's view of the boarding house as emblem-

atic of an entire American society "cemented by no tie, endeared by no connection, which choice did not bring together, and which the slightest motive would break asunder" (219–220).

20. Trollope, *Domestic Manners of the Americans*: 41.

21. Trollope, *Domestic Manners of the Americans*: 20.

22. Tyack, *George Ticknor*: 206.

23. Howells, *Literary Friends*: 101.

24. Warren, *John Collins Warren*: II, 257.

25. "Jonathan Edwards," in *Pages from an Old Volume of Life*: 384. Holmes' antipathy to Calvinism is standardly traced to his father's experience as a Congregational minister. The controversy in which Abiel Holmes was dismissed as minister of the First Congregational Church of Cambridge is recounted in detail in Tilton, 43–49. The issue had less to do with the Rev. Dr. Holmes' own religious opinions—"We are happy to testify," wrote the parish Council that called for his dismissal, "that our impressions of his course during the peaceful state of this society are associated with the most interesting and honorable views of his ministerial character and the Christian spirit. We sympathize with him under his trials" (Tilton: 47)—than with the demand of the *Boston Recorder*, backed by the fiery Calvinist Lyman Beecher, that ministers of "liberal" tendency no longer be permitted to give guest or "exchange" sermons in churches previously associated with an uncompromising Calvinist orthodoxy. Abiel Holmes had long been in the habit of carrying on the traditional "exchange of pulpits" with neighboring clergymen without regard to matters of doctrinal orthodoxy. When he abruptly altered his policy under pressure of Beecher's campaign, a substantial number of parishioners revolted, demanding a return to "that liberal system of professional exchanges" that had permitted them to listen to sermons delivered in the spirit of what would shortly become famous as Boston Unitarianism. It was, specifically, Abiel Holmes' refusal to comply that led to his dismissal.

26. Kennedy, *Holmes*: 130–131.

27. See Conor Cruise O'Brien, *The Long Affair*, and Dowling, *Literary Federalism*.

28. Arnold, *Memoir*: 74–75.

29. *Autocrat of the Breakfast Table*: 78.

30. *Autocrat of the Breakfast Table*: 2.

31. James Jackson, Sr., *Memoir*: 49–50.

32. Monsieur,

    J'ai l'honneur de vous annoncer que la Societé médicale d'Observation vous a admis au nombre de ses membres, à l'unanimité des suffrages.

    Veuillez agrier Monsieur l'assurance de ma consideration distingué

                        Le Secretaire J. Bizot

    Paris 16 Sept. 1834" (HCHL).

33. *Autocrat of the Breakfast Table*: 216–217.

34. *Autocrat of the Breakfast Table*: 280.

35. James Jackson, Sr., *Memoir*: 81.

36. Morse, *Life and Letters*: I, 100.

37. *Autocrat of the Breakfast Table*: 193.

38. *Professor at the Breakfast Table*: 244.

39. *Autocrat of the Breakfast Table*: 125.

40. "The Medical Profession in Massachusetts," in *Medical Essays*: 357.

41. *Professor at the Breakfast Table*: 247.

42. *Professor at the Breakfast Table*: 119.

43. "Jonathan Edwards." In *Pages from an Old Volume of Life*: 370.

44. "Jonathan Edwards." In *Pages from an Old Volume of Life*: 372. The quote is from Edwards's "The Great Christian Doctrine of Original Sin Defended."

45. "Jonathan Edwards." in *Pages from an Old Volume of Life*: 372–373.

46. "Jonathan Edwards." in *Pages from an Old Volume of Life*: 386.

47. "Jonathan Edwards," in *Pages from an Old Volume of Life*: 390.

48. HCHL: OWH personal notebook.

49. *Professor at the Breakfast Table*: 116.

50. *Professor at the Breakfast Table*: 116

51. HCHL: Lowell to OWH, 19 December 1858.

52. *Professor at the Breakfast Table*: 83.

53. *Professor at the Breakfast Table*: "Spiritual republicanism": Holmes, *Ralph Waldo Emerson*: 36.

54. *Professor at the Breakfast Table*: 105.

55. *Professor at the Breakfast Table*: *Professor*: 13.

56. "Democracy of ghosts": Nabokov. *Pnin*, Ch. 5.

57. *Professor at the Breakfast Table*: 12–13.

58. *Professor at the Breakfast Table*: 199.

59. *Poet at the Breakfast Table*: 83.

60. *Professor at the Breakfast Table*: 199.

61. *Professor at the Breakfast Table*: 256.

62. "Border Lines," in *Medical Essays*: 236.

63. *Autocrat of the Breakfast Table*: 29.

64. Kennedy, *Holmes*: 257.

65. Browne's remark occurs in a letter advising a young friend on a program of medical reading ("Read Fallopius, Aquapendente, Paraeus, Vigo, etc."): "Be sure you make yourself master of Dr. Harvey's piece *De Circu. Sang.*, which discovery I prefer to that of Columbus." Endicott, *The Prose of Sir Thomas Browne*: 497.

66. Browne, *Religio Medici*: 42.

67. *Professor at the Breakfast Table*: 58–59.

68. "Border Lines,"in *Medical Essays*: 236.

69. *Professor at the Breakfast Table*: 50.

70. Browne, *Religio Medici*: 19.

71. *Poet at the Breakfast Table*: 106–107.

72. Milton, *Paradise Lost*: II, 146–150.

73. Browne, *Religio Medici*: 45.

74. "Border Lines," in *Medical Essays*: 211.

75. "The Medical Profession in Massachusetts," in *Medical Essays*: 364.

76. Cited by Browne in *Religio Medici*: 28. Verse translation: John Wilmot, Earl of Rochester. *The Latter End of the Chorus of the Second Act of Seneca's Troas, Translated*. In *Poems by John Wilmot, Earl of Rochester*. Ed. Vivian de Sola Pinto. (Cambridge: Harvard University Press, 1953): 49.

77. Browne, *Religio Medici*: 51.

78. "The Medical Profession in Massachusetts," in *Medical Essays*: 365.

79. "The Pulpit and the Pew," in *Pages from an Old Volume of Life*: 414.

80. "Mechanism inThought and Morals," in *Pages from an Old Volume of Life*: 262.

81. *Professor at the Breakfast Table*: 177.

82. *Autocrat of the Breakfast Table*: 278.

83. Kennedy, *Holmes*: 97.

84. In *The Autocrat*, Holmes describes the Saturday Club as "strung like a harp, with about a dozen ringing intelligences, each answering to some chord of the macrocosm. They do well to dine together once in a while. A dinner-party made up of such elements is the last triumph of civilization over barbarism" (64).

85. *Poet at the Breakfast Table*: 48.

86. *The Poet at the Breakfast Table*: 58.

87. *Poet at the Breakfast Table*: 59.

88. *Poet at the Breakfast Table*: 136.

89. *Poet at the Breakfast Table*: 321.

90. *Poet at the Breakfast Table*: 321-22.

91. Howells, *Literary Friends*: 145

92. *Poet at the Breakfast Table*: vii.

Works Cited and Selective Bibliography

Ackerknecht, Erwin H. *Medicine at the Paris Hospital, 1794–1848* (Baltimore: Johns Hopkins Press, 1967).

Albury, W. R. "Corvisart and Broussais: Human Individuality and Medical Dominance." In Hannaway and La Berge, *Constructing Paris Medicine.*

Anderson, Quentin. "Henry James's Cultural Office." In *Prospects: The Annual of American Cultural Studies.* Ed. Jack Salzman (Cambridge, England: Cambridge University Press, 1983).

Arnold, Howard Payson. *Memoir of Jonathan Mason Warren, M.D.* (Boston: privately printed, 1886).

Bailyn, Bernard. *The Ideological Origins of the American Revolution* (Cambridge: Harvard University Press, 1967).

Bartlett, Elisha. *A Discourse on the Times, Character and Writings of Hippocrates* (New York: H. Baillière, 1832).

Bartlett, Elisha. *An Enquiry into the Degree of Certainty in Medicine* (Philadelphia: Les and Blanchard, 1848).

Bartlett, Elisha. *An Essay on the Philosophy of Medical Science* (Philadelphia: Lea and Blanchard, 1844).

Bartholow, Roberts. *A Practical Treatise on Materia Medica and Therapeutics* (New York: Appleton, 1884).

Bigelow, Henry J. *Medical Education in America* (Cambridge, Mass.: Welch, Biglow, and Company, 1871).

Bigelow, Henry Jacob. *Science and Success: A Valedictory Address Delivered to the Medical Graduates of Harvard University . . . March 9, 1859.*

Bigelow, Jacob. *Nature and Disease* (Boston: Ticknor and Fields, 1854).

Bonnett, Thomas Neville. *Becoming a Physician: Medical Education in Britain, France, Germany, and the United States, 1750–1945* (New York: Oxford University Press, 1995).

Bowditch, Henry I. *Brief Memories of Louis and Some of His Contemporaries in the Parisian School of Medicine of Forty Years Ago* (Boston: John Wilson and Son, 1872.)

Bowditch, Vincent Y., ed. *Life and Correspondence of Henry Ingersoll Bowditch,* 2 vols. (Boston: Houghton Mifflin and Company, 1902).

Braunstein, Jean-François. *Broussais et le matérialisme: médecine et philosophie au XIXe siècle* (Paris: Meridiens Klincksieck, 1986).

Brockliss, L. W. B. "Before the Clinic: French Medical Teaching in the Eighteenth Century." In Hannaway and La Berge, *Constructing Paris Medicine.*

Brockliss, L. W. B. *"L'enseignment médical et la Révolution: essai de réévaluation."* Histoire de l'education 42 (1989): 79-110.

Brooks, Van Wyck, *The Flowering of New England* (New York: Dutton, 1952).

Broussais, F. J. V. *Examen des doctriens médicales. 2 vols.* (Paris: Mequignon-Marvis, 1821).

Browne, Sir Thomas. *Religio Medici.* In *The Prose of Sir Thomas Browne.* Ed. Norman J. Endicott (New York: Doubleday & Company, 1967).

Buchan, William. *Domestic Medicine: or, the Family Physician.* 2nd American ed. (Philadelphia: Joseph Crukshank, 1774).

Burr, Anna R. *Weir Mitchell: His Life and Letters* (New York: Duffield, 1929).

Bynum, W. F. *Science and the Practice of Medicine in the Nineteenth Century* (Cambridge, England: Cambridge University Press, 1994).

Carlyle, Thomas. *The Correspondence of Thomas Carlyle and Ralph Waldo Emerson* [see Norton, Charles Eliot].

Cook, Harold J. "Boerhaave and the Flight from Reason in Medicine." *Bulletin of the History of Medicine* 74:2 (2000): 221–240.

Currier, Thomas Franklin, and Eleanor M. Tilton. *A Bibliography of Oliver Wendell Holmes* (New York: NYU Press, 1953).

Curtis, George William, ed. *The Correspondence of John Lothrop Motley.* 2 vols. (New York: Harper and Brothers, 1889).

Daniels, George H. *American Science in the Age of Jackson* (New York: Columbia University Press, 1968).

Delaporte, François. *Disease and Civilization: The Cholera in Paris, 1832.* Trans. Arthur Goldhammer (Cambridge: MIT Press, 1986).

Delaunay, Paul. *D'une révolution à l'autre, 1789–1848: l'évolution des théories et de la practique médicales* (Paris: Editions Hippocrate, 1949).

Dowling, William C. "Dr. Holmes and the Paris Medical Revolution: The Inaugural Lecture on Anatomy and Physiology at Dartmouth Medical School." *Dartmouth College Library Bulletin* 42 (April 2002): 60–11.

Dowling, William C. *The Epistolary Moment: The Poetics of the Eighteenth-Century Verse Epistle* (Princeton: Princeton University Press, 1991).

Dowling, William C. *Literary Federalism in the Age of Jefferson* (Columbia: University of South Carolina Press, 1999).

Dubos, Rene and Jean. *The White Plague: Tuberculosis, Man and Society* (Boston: Little, Brown and Company, 1952).

Duffin, Jacalyn. *To See with a Better Eye: A Life of R. T. H. Laennec.* (Princeton: Princeton University Press, 1998).

Duffin, Jacalyn. *History of Medicine* (Toronto: University of Toronto Press, 1999).

Ellis, Harold. *A History of the Bladder Stone* (Oxford: Blackwell, 1969).

Emerson, Ralph Waldo. *The Correspondence of Thomas Carlyle and Ralph Waldo Emerson* [see Norton, Charles Eliot].

Emerson, Ralph Waldo. *Journals, Journals of Ralph Waldo Emerson.* Ed. Edward Waldo Emerson and Waldo Emerson Forbes. 10 vols. (Boston: Houghton, Mifflin and Company, 1909-1914).

Estes, J. Worth. *Dictionary of Protopharmacology: Therapeutic Practices, 1700–1850* (Canton, MA: Watson Publishing, 1990).

Fields, Annie. *Authors and Friends* (Boston: Houghton, Mifflin and Company, 1896).

Forbes, John. *A Treatise on Diseases of the Chest and on Mediate Auscultation* (London: T. and G. Underwood, 1827). [Translation and abridgement of Laennec's *De l'auscultation médiate*].

Foucault, Michel. *Naissance de la clinique* (Paris: Galien, 1963).

Frazee, L. J. *The Medical Student in Europe* (Maysville, Kentucky: Richard U. Collins, 1849).

Fye, W. Bruce. *The Development of American Physiology: Scientific Medicine in the Nineteenth Century* (Baltimore: Johns Hopkins, 1987).

Galignani's New Paris Guide, or, Stranger's Companion Through the French Metropolis, 14th ed. (Paris: A. & W. Galignani, 1826).

Gardner, Augustus Kinsley. *Old Wine in New Bottles; or, Spare Hours of a Student in Paris* (New York: C.S. Francis & Co, 1848).

Gelfand, Toby. *Professionalizing Modern Medicine: Paris Surgeons and Medical Science and Institutions in the Eighteenth Century* (Westport, Conn.: Greenwood Press, 1980).

Gibian, Peter. *Oliver Wendell Holmes and the Culture of Conversation* (Cambridge and New York: Cambridge University Press, 2001).

Gibson, William. *Rambles in Europe in 1839. With sketches of Prominent Surgeons, Physicians, Medical Schools, Hospitals, Literary Personages, Scenery, Etc.* (Philadelphia: Lea and Blanchard, 1841).

Hacking, Ian. *Rewriting the Soul: Multiple Personality and the Sciences of Memory* (Princeton: Princeton University Press, 1995).

Hale, Susan. *The Life and Letters of Thomas Gold Appleton* (New York: D. Appleton and Co., 1885).

Haller, John S. *The People's Doctors: Samuel Thomson and the American Botanical Movement, 1790–1860* (Carbondale: Southern Illinois University Press, 2000).

Hannaway, Caroline, and La Berge, Anne, eds. *Constructing Paris Medicine* (Amsterdam: Editions Rodopi, 1998).

Head, Sir Francis. *A Faggot of French Sticks, or, Paris in 1851* (New York: George Putnam, 1852).

Holmes, Oliver Wendell. *Boylston Prize Dissertations for the Years 1836 and 1837* (Boston: Charles C. Little and James Brown, 1838).

Holmes, Oliver Wendell. *Soundings from the Atlantic* (Boston: James R. Osgood, 1872).

Holmes, Oliver Wendell. *The Writings of Oliver Wendell Holmes.* 13 vols. (Boston: Houghton, Mifflin and Company, 1891).

Holmes, Urban Tigner. *Daily Living in the Twelfth Century, Based on the Observations of Alexander Neckam in London and Paris* (Madison: University of Wisconsin Press, 1964.)

Houghton, Walter E. *The Victorian Frame of Mind, 1830–1870* (New Haven: Yale University Press, 1957).

Howe, Mark De Wolfe. *The Atlantic Monthly and Its Makers* (Boston: Atlantic Monthly Press, 1919).

Howe, Mark DeWolfe. *Justice Oliver Wendell Holmes: The Shaping Years, 1841–1847*, 2 vols. (Cambridge: Harvard University Press, 1957).

Howe, Mark DeWolfe. *Holmes of the Breakfast Table* (London: Oxford University Press, 1939).

Howells, W. D. *Literary Friends and Acquaintance*, ed. David F. Hiatt and Edwin H. Cady (Bloomington: Indiana University Press, 1968).

Hoyt, Edwin P. *The Improper Bostonian: Dr. Oliver Wendell Holmes* (New York: Morrow, 1979).

Jackson, James, Sr. *A Memoir of James Jackson, Jr.* (Boston: privately printed, 1863).

Jacyna, Stephen. "'Au lit des malades': A.F. Chomel's clinic at the Charité, 1828-29." *Medical History* 33 (1989): 420–449.

Jacyna, Stephen. *Philosophical Whigs: Medicine, Science and Citizenship in Edinburgh, 1789–1848* (London: Routledge, 1994).

Jewson, N. D. "The Disappearance of the Sick-Man from Medical Cosmology, 1770-1870." *Sociology* 10 (1978): 225–244.

Johnson, Samuel. *Lives of the English Poets*. Ed. George Birkbeck Hill. 3 vols. (Oxford: Clarendon Press, 1895).

Jones, Russell M. "American Doctors in Paris, 1820–1861: A Statistical Profile," *Journal of the History of Medicine and Allied Sciences* 25 (1970): 142–157.

Jones, Russell M. "American Doctors and the Parisian Medical World, 1830-1840." *Bulletin of the History of Medicine* 47 (1793): 40–85, 177–204.

Jones, Russell M. *The Parisian Education of an American Surgeon: Letters of Jonathan Mason Warren, 1832–1835* (Philadelphia: American Philosophical Society, 1978).

Kaufman, Martin. *Homeopathy in America: The Rise and Fall of a Medical Heresy* (Baltimore: Johns Hopkins University Press, 1971).

Keel, Othmar. *La généalogie de l'histopathologie* (Paris: J. Vrin, 1979).

Keel, Othmar. "Was Anatomical and Tissue Pathology a Product of the Paris Clinical School?" In Hannaway and La Berge, *Constructing Paris Medicine*.

Kelly, Howard A., and Burrage, Walter L., eds. *Dictionary of American Medical Biography* (Boston: Milford House, 1971).

Kennedy, William Sloane. *Oliver Wendell Holmes: Poet, Littérateur, Scientist* (Boston: S.E. Cassino & Co., 1883).

Kerber, Linda K. *Federalists in Dissent: Imagery and Ideology in Jeffersonian America* (Ithaca, N.Y.: Cornell University Press, 1970).

Ketcham, Michael G. *Transparent Designs: Reading, Performance, and Form in the "Spectator" Papers* (Athens: University of Georgia Press, 1835).

King, Lester S. *American Medicine Comes of Age, 1840-1920* (Chicago: American Medical Association, 1984).

King, Lester S. *The Medical World of the Eighteenth Century* (Chicago: University of Chicago Press, 1958.) Rpt. Robert E. Krieger Publishing, 1971.

Kohl, Frederick. *The Politics of Individualism: Parties and the American Character in the Jacksonian Era* (New York: Oxford University Press, 1989).

Laennec, R. T. H. *De l'auscultation médiate* (Paris: Brusson et Chaudé, 1819).

Lesch, John E. *Science and Medicine in France: The Emergence of Experimental Physiology, 1790–1855* (Cambridge: Harvard University Press, 1984).

Long, Esmond. *A History of Pathology*. (Baltimore: Williams & Wilkins, 1928).

Louis, P. C. A. *Researches on the Effects of Bloodletting*. Trans. C. G. Putnam. (Boston: Hilliard, Gray, and Company, 1836).

Louis, P. C. A. *Researches on Phthisis*. Trans. Walter Hayle Walshe (London: Sydenham Society, 1844).

Louis, P. C. A. *Examen de l'examen de M. Broussais, relativement à la Phthisie et à L'affection Typhoïde* (Paris: J. B. Ballière, 1834).

Lowell, James Russell. *The Round Table* (Boston: Gorham, 1913).

Maulitz, Russell C. *Morbid Appearances: The Anatomy of Pathology in the Early Nineteenth Century* (Cambridge: Cambridge University Press, 1987).

Meding, Henri. *Paris médicale: vademecum des médecins étrangers*. 2 vols. (Paris: J.B. Balière, 1852–53).

Miller, Perry. *The Raven and the Whale* (New York: Harcourt Brace, 1956).

Montaigne, Michel Eyquem de. *The Essays of Michael Lord of Montaigne*. Trans. John Florio. 3 vols. (London: J. M. Dent, 1928).

Mordell, Albert. *The Autocrat's Miscellanies* (New York: Twayne, 1989).

Morse, John T., Jr. *Life and Letters of Oliver Wendell Holmes*, 2 vols. (New York: Chelsea House, 1980).

Motley, John Lothrop. *Correspondence* [see Curtis, George William].

Mott, Valentine. *Travels in Europe and the East* (New York: Harper & Brothers, 1842).

Nabokov, Vladimir. *Pnin* (New York: Random House, 1953).

Norton, Charles Eliot, ed. *The Correspondence of Thomas Carlyle and Ralph Waldo Emerson*, 2 vols. (Boston: Ticknor and Company, 1888).

Nissenbaum, Stephen. *Sex, Diet, and Debility in Jacksonian America: Sylvester Graham and Health Reform* (Westport, Conn: Greenwood Press, 1980).

Nuland, Sherwin B. *Doctors: The Biography of Medicine* (New York: Vintage, 1988).

Nuland, Sherwin B. *How We Die: Reflections on Life's Final Chapter* (New York: Random House, 1993).

O'Brien, Conor Cruise. *The Long Affair: Thomas Jefferson and the French Revolution, 1785–1800* (Chicago: University of Chicago Press, 1996).

Osler, William. *An Alabama Student: and Other Biographical Essays* (London: Henry Frowde, 1909).

Paley, William. *Natural Theology: or, Evidences of the Existence and Attributes of the Deity, Collected from the Appearances of Nature* (Boston: Gould and Lincoln, 1860).

Parker, Theodore. *The Nebraska Question* (Boston: Benjamin B. Mussey & Co., 1854).

Pocock, J. G. A. *The Machiavellian Moment* (Princeton: Princeton University Press, 1975).

Putnam, Constance E. *Improve, Perfect, & Perpetuate: Dr. Nathan Smith and Early American Medical Education* (Hanover: University Press of New England, 1998).

Ramsey, Matthew. *Professional and Popular Medicine in France, 1770–1830: The Social World of Medical Practice* (New York: Cambridge University Press, 1988).

Rees, Robert A., and Earl N. Harbert, eds. *Fifteen American Authors Before 1900: Bibliographic Essays on Research and Criticism* (Madison: University of Wisconsin Press, 1971).

Rosen, George. "The Philosophy of Ideology and the Emergence of Modern Medicine in France." *Bulletin of the History of Medicine* 20 (1946): 328–339.

Rothstein, William G. *American Physicians in the Nineteenth Century: From Sects to Science* (Baltimore: Johns Hopkins University Press, 1972.)

Sartin, Jeffrey S., and Perry, Harold O. "From mercury to malaria to penicillin: The history of the treatment of syphilis at the Mayo Clinic, 1916–1955." *Journal of the American Academy of Dermatology* 32 (1995): 255–261.

Sellers, Charles. *The Market Revolution: Jacksonian America, 1815–1836* (New York: Oxford University Press, 1991).

Shryock, Richard H. *The Development of Modern Medicine: An Interpretation of the Social and Scientific Factors Involved* (Madison: University of Wisconsin Press, 1979).

Shryock, Richard Harrison. *Medical Licensing in America, 1650–1965* (Baltimore: Johns Hopkins UP, 1967).

Smith, Dale C. "Gerhard's Distinction between Typhoid and Typhus and its Reception in America, 1833–1860." *Bulletin of the History of Medicine* 34 (1980):368–383.

Smith, Henry H. *A Professional Visit to London and Paris* (Philadelphia: T.K. & P.G. Collins, 1855).

Staum, Martin. *Cabanis: Enlightenment and Medical Philosophy in the French Republic* (Princeton: Princeton University Press, 1980).

Stewart, F. Campbell. *Eminent French Surgeons, with a Historical and Statistical Account of the Hospitals of Paris* (Buffalo: A. Burke, 1845).

Thomson, Samuel. *New Guide to Health; or, Botanic Family Physician* (Boston: J.Q. Adams, 1833).

Tilanus, C. B. *Surgery A Hundred Years Ago. Extracts from the Diary of Dr. C.B. Tilanus, Afterwards Professor of Surgery at the University of Amsterdam*, ed. H. T. Deelman. Trans. Joseph Bles. (London: Geoffrey Bles: Suffolk St., Pall Mall, 1925).

Tiles, Mary. *Bachelard: Science and Objectivity* (Cambridge, England: Cambridge University Press, 1984).

Tilton, Eleanor M. *Amiable Autocrat: A Biography of Dr. Oliver Wendell Holmes* (New York: Farrar, Straus and Giroux, 1978).

Tocqueville, Alexis de. *Democracy in America*, 2 vols. Ed. Phillips Bradley. Trans. Henry Reeve, rev. Francis Bowen. (New York: Alfred A. Knopf, 1973).

Trollope, Frances. *Domestic Manners of the Americans*, ed. Pamela Neville-Sington (London: Penguin Books, 1997).

Trollope, Frances. *Paris and the Parisians in 1835*, 2 vols. (Paris: A. and W. Galignani and Co, 1836).

Tyack, David B. *George Ticknor and the Boston Brahmins* (Cambridge: Harvard University Press, 1967).

Warner, John Harley. *Against the Spirit of System: The French Impulse in Nineteenth-Century American Medicine* (Princeton: Princeton University Press, 1998).

Warner, John Harley. "Paradigm Lost or Paradise Declining? American Physicians and the 'Dead End' of the Paris Clinical School." In Hannaway and La Berge, *Constructing Paris Medicine*.

Warner, John Harley. *The Therapeutic Perspective: Medical Practice, Knowledge, and Identity in America, 1820–1885* (Cambridge: Harvard University Press, 1986).

Warren, Edward, ed. *The Life of John Collins Warren, M.D., Compiled Chiefly from His Autobiography and Journals*, 2 vols. (Boston: Ticknor and Fields, 1860).

Warren, Jonathan Mason. *Letters* [see Jones, Russell M.].

Weiss, John. *The Life and Correspondence of Theodore Parker*, 2 vols. (New York, D. Appleton, 1864).

Wendell, Barrett. *A Literary History of America* (New York: Scribners, 1900).

Whitney, Daniel H. *The Family Physician: or Every Man His Own Doctor* (New York: N. and J. White, 1834).

Williams, Elizabeth. *The Physical and the Moral: Anthropology, Physiology, and Philosophical Medicine in France, 1730–1850* (Cambridge, England: Cambridge University Press, 1994).

Index

108; skepticism about vox populi quoted by OWH, 159n88
Enfants Malades (hospital), 9
English Humourists, vii
Enlightenment materialism, xv, 6, 130
epistemological rupture, x. See also *coupure épistémologique*
erysipelas (*streptococcus pyogenes*): as postoperative infection, 22; and puerperal fever, 92, 94
erythrocyte, 128

Family Physician, The, 106
Fielding, Henry, vii
Fifth Monarchy Men, 104
Forbes, John, 33, 40–43
Foucault, Michel, 12
Fourcroy, Antoine François, 7–8; concept of the teaching hospital, 9
Freneau, Philip, 140
Frère Côme, 20, 22
Fuller, Margaret, 140

Galen, 3–4, 7, 10, 12, 50, 127. *See also* humoral medicine
Galileo, 127
Gardner, Augustus: 16, 87; on Paris dissection facilities, xi; on the coarseness of American society, 8; on *concours* system as democratic ideal, 11
Gerhard, William, 32, 41, 46, 54; distinction between typhus and typhoid fever, 77
Gibian, Peter, 140
Gibson, William: *Rambles in Europe*, 148n3
Goldsmith, Oliver, vii
Gosse, Edmund, 142
Green, John Orne, 113
Gutenberg, Johann, 5

Hacking, Ian, 145n13
Hahnemann, Samuel, 101–102, 131
Haller, John, 143
Hamlet, 134
Hannaway, Caroline, 138
Harvey, William, 13, 127–128; *De motu cordis*, 12

Hawthorne, Nathaniel, 116, 140
Helvetius (Helvétius, Claude Arien), ix, 84
hemoglobin, 127–128
Hempstead, G. S. B., 64
Herbert, Earl N., 139, 142
heroic treatment, 62, 71
Hersey, Thomas, 105
Hippocrates, 6, 12, 38, 41, 127; forbids cutting for the stone, 18
Hodge, Hugh, L., 95–98
Holbach, Paul Henri, Baron d', viii, 6, 44, 84
Holmes, Abiel, 132; controversy surrounding his dismissal as pastor of First Congregational Church, 160n25
Holmes, John (brother of OWH), 31
Holmes, Oliver Wendell, Sr.: as *Atlantic* contributor, vii; *Mechanism in Thought and Morals* and French materialism, x; metaphysics of consciousness, x, 54, 86, 126; Boylston Prize essays, xi, 40, 50–52; Paris medical studies and repudiation of Calvinism, xiv; science as modern form of divine revelation, xiv, 87, 111; *religio medici*, xv; final address to Harvard medical students, 1, 55; account of humoral theory, 4; on Velpeau and *concours* system, 11; regional anatomy as "geology of the body," 15; on Paris anatomical dissection, 16; replaces J. C. Warren as Parkman Professor at Harvard, 27; offered Chair of Surgery at University of Maryland, 29; arrival in Paris, 28; facility in learning languages, 30; essay on puerperal fever, 32; lodgings at 55 rue M. Le Prince, 32; persona in *Autocrat* influenced by theatricality of Parisian medical teaching, 48; on scientific ignorance, 50; cites "MS notes" to Chomel's lectures, 52; receives M.D., 52; on persistence of bloodletting as remedy, 64; on Benjamin Rush and Jeffersonian democracy, 66; *post hoc ergo propter hoc* as origin of medical error, 75; essay on puerperal fever modeled on Louis's

Holmes, Oliver Wendell, Sr. *(continued)*
Examen, 69; publication of *Puerperal Fever as a Private Pestilence,* 96; puerperal fever paper delivered to Society for Medical Improvement, 91; discovers mode of double enunciation in puerperal fever essay, 99; medical doctrine as civic discourse, 101; opposition to Jacksonian medicine, 107; American republic as "chosen home of minorities," 109; "this infinite, instantaneous consciousness in which the soul's being consists," 112; stream-of-consciousness style, 113; detestation of Calvinist doctrine of predestination, 116; mentions puerperal fever controversy in *Poet at the Breakfast Table,* 120; on Calvinist doctrine of infant damnation, 121; as spiritual physician, 127; science as based in human consciousness, 128; on microscopy and the birth of cell biology, 156n4
homeopathy, 74, 80, 82, 100, 107; doctrine of infinitesimal doses, 102; analogy of infinitesimal doses with vaccination, 103; as preserving patients from heroic remedies, 124
Homer, 113
Hospital of Necker, 3
Hôtel Dieu (hospital), 7–8
Howe, Mark Antony DeWolfe, 141
Howells, William Dean, xiv–xv, 99, 116; OWH as moralist, 134
humoral theory, 3–4, 43, 54, 62, 64, 73
Hunterian Museum (London), 18
Huxley, Thomas Henry, ix, 131

Innate Depravity, xiv
inter taedia et labores, 34
ipecacuanha, 63

Jackson, Andrew: as "second Jefferson," 78; Jacksonian medicine ("people's doctors" and Jacksonian democracy) 54, 101, 115; political opposition to medical licensing, 107; Jacksonian political ideology, 11, 56, 104, 115; 109; as encouraging medical

charlatanism, 79; and economic individualism, 77; as indiscriminate populism, 113
Jackson, James, Jr., 2, 25, 28–29, 32, 41, 46, 49, 54–55 , 60, 66–67, 70, 77; difficulty of examining patients during Chomel's clinical rounds, 31; death as symbolic episode, 59–60
Jackson, James, Sr., 60, 68, 71, 118; pure medical research unthinkable in U.S., 57; *Memoir* of son issues warning against heroic practice, 67; recommends *méthode expectante* and numerical method, 70; letter to Louis, 119
Jacobin party, 117
Jacyna, L. S., 78, 146n16
jalap, 63, 67
Jardin des Plantes, ix, 29, 87
Jeffersonian ideology, 61
Jenner, Edward, 102, 105
Johnson, Samuel, 113, 127
Jones, Russell M., 138

Kant, Immanuel, 112, 133
Kaufman, Martin, 108
Keel, Othmar, 137–138
Kennedy, William Sloane, xv, 96, 117, 127, 142
King, Lester, 57
Kingsley, Charles, 110
Knepfler, Nathan, 65
Kohl, Frederick: Andrew Jackson as "second Jefferson," 155
Kuhn, Thomas, 145n13

La Pitié (hospital), 25, 29, 46, 55, 71, 77, 91, 134
La Berge, Anne, 138
La Charité (hospital), xi, 11, 49, 84. See also *école de La Charité;* school of La Charité
La Mettrie, Julien Offroy de, ix, 6, 44
Laennec, René Théophile Hyacinthe, xi, 5, 10, 12–13, 30–31, 33, 35, 44, 47, 49, 52, 69, 77, 108, 137; discovery of auscultation, 36; teaches in Latin, 36; discovery of pectoriloquy, 37; description of tubercular excava-

Thomson, Samuel, 41, 64, 74, 104, 104; denounces regularly educated physicians as "aristocracy," 106
Thoreau, Henry David, 80, 116
Ticknor, George, 81, 116
Tilanus, C. B., 20–21, 23
Tiles, Mary, 145n13
Tilton, Eleanor M., 141
Tocqueville, Alexis de, 59–60, 77; on American worship of wealth, 56; on profit motive in American society, 58–59; on American pressure to mass conformity, 79; on American contempt for intellectual pursuits, 80; on American pressure to conform to public opinion, 155n90
Total Depravity, 121–122
Transcendentalism, 80
Tremont Medical School, 158n158
trilabe, 3
Trois Frères Provençaux, 117
Trollope, Frances, 79, 119, 132; boarding house as symbol of Jacksonian democracy, 115–116, 160n19; on medical mountebanks in nineteenth-century Paris, 155
tubercular excavations, xi

ubi tres medici, duo athei, 130
Underwood, Francis H., vii, 142
unguentum armarium, 101
Unitarianism, 84
University of Pennsylvania, 63
Ussher, James, Archbishop of Armagh, 125–126

Val de Grâce (hospital), 44–45, 47
Vanity Fair (Thackeray), vii
Vassar College, viii
Velpeau, Armand, 2, 11, 58, 89; as symbol of the merits of the *concours* system, 151n11
Vicq d'Azyr, Félix, 7–8
Victorian religious anxiety, 110

Vienna Hospital, 92
Virchow, Rudolf, xiii, xiv, 71, 128
Virgil, 113
vis medicatrix naturae, xiii–x, 25, 37, 43, 76–77, 81, 84, 88–89, 91, 103; as antidote to New England theology, 89; as evidence of divine benevolence, 131
Voltaire, (François Marie Arouet), 84

Warner, John Harley, x, 15, 44, 56, 62, 79, 139, 143
Warren, Edward, 77, 116, 139
Warren, John Collins, 2, 17, 25, 66, 139; account of *concours* system, 10; visits Paris to study with Louis, 26; account of grave-robbing by Harvard medical students, 15; performs first operation under anesthesia, 26
Warren, Mason (Jonathan Mason), 2, 10, 16, 25, 28, 32, 55–56, 71, 76, 81, 115, 117, 138; account of Civiale's procedure, 2; description of Civiale's procedure, 17; practices Civiale's procedure, 22; describes Lisfranc's regimen of postoperative bleeding, 23; asks father for additional Paris year to study with Louis, 25; as pioneer in plastic surgery, 26; describes operation by Roux, 29; difficulty learning French, 30; description of subcrepitant rale, 42; on Louis's numerical method, 67
Wendell, Barrett, 141
Wesley, Samuel, 104
Wheatley, Phillis, 140
Whitman, Walt, 140
Whitney, Daniel H., 106
Wilde, Oscar, 13
Williams, Charles J. B., 40, 43
Winthrop, John, 90

yellow fever, 61
Yellowplush Papers (Thackeray), vii